LOVING

TRUTHS ABOUT SEX NO ONE TOLD YOU

Emmanuel Williams

ISBN: 1-4196-9152-X

ISBN-13: 9781419691522

Visit www.booksurge.com to order additional copies.

LOVING

Truths about sex no one told you

Acknowledgements

My thanks are due to Salamah Pope, without whose encouragement this book would never have been written.

I would also like to say Thank You to all those men and women who trusted me with accounts of their experiences. I've changed their names to protect their privacy.

My gratitude also goes to the Trustees of the Subud Talent Bank for their support.

LOVING

IS DEDICATED WITH LOVE TO MY WIFE AMELIA

"America doesn't have clearly defined and universally accepted rules about sexuality. We live in a pluralistic society with contradictory sexual paradigms."

Mary Pipher, *Reviving Ophelia*

"...there is a hole in our dialog about sexuality. The idea is that it's a very free time, but it's also a very scary time."

Martabel Waserman, editor, *H Bomb, Harvard sex magazine*

"We live with the sexual revolution, and the reaction against the sexual revolution. We struggle with both the desire to... do whatever we feel like after two drinks on a Saturday night, and to be bounded by the rules; and it's in the uneasiness and confusion of this struggle that most of us love and are loved."

Katie Roiphe, *Last Night in Paradise*

"Sex, when it is a vehicle for love, is holy. Sex without love is dangerous. It leads to pain and some level of emotional destruction, whether consciously experienced or not. Sex should be a deepening of communication, not a substitute for it."

Marianne Williamson, *Illuminata*

"When you're young you think that sex is the culmination of intimacy. Later, you discover that it's barely the beginning."

Peter Hoeg, *Miss Smilla's Feeling of Snow*

"Love is not the result of adequate sexual satisfaction, but sexual happiness - even the knowledge of the so-called sexual techniques - is the result of love."

Erich Fromm, *The Art of Loving*

"We have a habit of talking about sex as merely physical, and yet nothing has more soul…. Even if sex is loveless, empty or manipulative, still it has strong repercussions in the soul, and bad sexual experiences leave a lasting, haunting impression."

Thomas Moore, *The Soul of Sex*

CONTENTS

Introduction I

How having sex affects us 1

Fields 15

Basic Level of Being 21

Invisible People 27

Sex in the Head 31

Being the Boss 45

The Choice 51

Romantic Love 57

What's right for me 65

Who am I? 75

The Vacuum 83

The Law of Cosmic Balance 97

Abortion 103

Celibacy 119

Making Babies 133

Conclusion 137

Appendix 141

Life Energies 143

Male and Female 155

References 167

Bibliography 171

INTRODUCTION

.... as so many people are having sex these days, people think it's just ordinary, normal. But the point is... you are making these decisions without having all the information! Because no one today knows about the spiritual consequences.
                                                    – Julia, Australia

Sex, I've realized, is *very very big*. It's a real mystery, up there with death, birth and God. This book is about sex, and I have to acknowledge at the start that I really don't know very much about it. Compared to what there is to be known, I mean. But I've discovered some truths about sex which I thought others might find interesting, even useful.

Most people have a few relationships, and then get married and stay faithful to their spouse. They seem to ride high and light through life, delivered from or resisting temptation when it whispers in their ear or indeed any of their organs. For others, the delights of sex are irresistible, and they may spend years on what Shakespeare so charmingly called "The primrose path of dalliance." I was a primrose path man for decades, following my bliss in blissful innocence. Eventually, after a series of experiences I'm about to recount, I realized that there's a lot more to sex than I'd ever suspected. However casually we treat it, sex, I discovered, is *never* casual. And if we don't respect it, sex can do us a great deal of harm.

I believe this to be a truth. But as I said, sex is a mystery, so when I express a "truth" about it I'm aware that what I'm saying is almost certainly incomplete. So please don't make a guru of me and believe everything I say. Take my words into your guts for a while and feel them out for yourself. Don't *think* about too much about it, and please try not to *react*. Don't get angry with me. I'm not judging you. Use your intuition. Test what I say against your own experience and what you've learnt from it. Try to respond rather than react.

My beliefs about sex arose out of a whole series of experiences, both outer and inner, and it seems right that I tell you about some of them so that you can see how I came to I think as I do.

For at least twenty years, through the 1960s and 70s, I was a lover of women. I was either seeking a relationship, involved in a relationship, or getting over a relationship. I did a lot of other things - I went to university, taught, traveled, wrote, played sports, enjoyed the natural world – particularly the coast - performed in a poetry-rock band called The Electric Robin and acted in community theater… but mostly I was spending time with, being in love with, making love with, or breaking up with, whoever was my current girl-friend. I wasn't promiscuous. I was a sexual romantic. One at a time - but who the one is, changes.

This is the lifestyle of characters in shows like 'Friends' and 'Seinfeld' and in the Woody Allen movie 'Annie Hall'. This was how most of my friends lived. I never wondered whether I was learning anything or growing inwardly, or even harming myself. Why should I? I was in a state of innocence.

Things went on like this until I was in my mid-thirties. I was living in a hippie commune in the West of England (I'm English by the way.) There came a day when, abuzz with some dubious substance, I climbed to the top of a tree and hung on there, holding onto one of the highest branches. It was autumn; all around me big trees were turning yellow and bronze, crimson and copper. The wind was gusting, and my treetop was swaying to and fro so that I had the blissful feeling that I was atop a tall mast on a schooner swinging through a sea of copper and gold.

I sensed that a phase of my life was ending and another was beginning. I gripped the trunk with my thighs, held my hands up to the sky and yelled: *"God, whatever you want of me, I accept it!"*

Next day a telegram arrived from a school principal I knew in London: "*I need you in my school. Please come.*"

So I traveled to London and visited her school. She wanted to take eight highly disruptive boys out of their regular classes, where they were creating chaos, give me a room, and have me work with them.

I'd made my promise to God. Now I had to keep it.

I said Okay.

I did this for eight months.

Those boys knocked the crap out of me. They "dismantled " me, to quote the Huckabees movie. They were so raw and needy that they stripped me down to my core, which was the only part of me they respected. One day I lost it and I threw a kid - Bennett - on the floor. He hurt his head. I took him to the principal's office, told her what had happened, left him with her and walked back to the classroom. The kids were very quiet. I sat at my desk and put my head on my arms. I felt like an ogre. I heard the door open. I heard whisperings, and rustlings. I didn't care what they were doing. I was near to tears. I felt some light papery object placed on my head. "Sir…" said Bennett's voice. I sat up and took the thing off my head. It was a crown. Written on it were the words:

YOU ARE THE KING

By the end of our time together I felt like I'd been forced through an industrial strength psyche-washing machine. I felt simultaneously grateful to the kids for all they'd given me - intense and difficult though our time together had been - and totally lost. I had no idea who I was or what I should do next. A close relationship I'd been having with an American woman ended. I felt a desperate need to go somewhere totally different, take stock, start again. My inner was yelling at me with increasing urgency: **"Get me out of here!"**

So then it was a question of where I should go. I threw the I Ching – something many of us did at the time – and got the message that I should go to a community where there were those who were older and wiser than myself. I'd been a Subud member for a while, then dropped out when things went crazy. I'd also become interested in Zen – something else many of us did at the time. So I had a choice: go to Cilandak, a Subud community near Jakarta, in Java, or go to a Zen monastery in Scotland. (You can look up Subud on the web.) Still too confused to trust myself with this decision I tossed a coin. Heads Cilandak, tails Scotland.

Shortly after this I flew to Jakarta. Got a taxi to Cilandak. I'd planned on staying a month or two. Recharge my psychic batteries, then come home and try to do better. The quick journey to enlightenment was a popular myth of the times. I immediately came down with amoebic dysentery and spent two weeks either lying in a hot little room out of my head with a high fever, or scurrying down the corridor to the "mandi" – the rest-room. I felt – if you'll pardon the expression – as though I was pouring out of myself. I saw my parents, my old lovers and my friends floating around my room

I V

like helium balloons, smiling encouragingly. I thought I might be dying. In a manner of speaking, I was.

As my fever cooled and I regained a degree of normal consciousness, I sensed that spiritually I was in a pretty bad way. I told everyone I met, with a kind of hysterical solemnity, that I had destroyed my soul. I kept thinking of piles of malodorous garbage. This was an uncomfortable phase. I prayed, urgently: "*Please God, if it's right for me to stay here, make it possible.*"

A few weeks later I landed a teaching job at a nearby international school. This was the first time I'd ever consciously prayed for something. The fact that my prayer was answered changed everything.

So there I was, a serial lover of women, suddenly placed in a very foreign culture, in a community with quite a strong spiritual atmosphere. I was - mainly through lack of opportunity - celibate. There were no drugs to be had. Three young women – one American, one English and one Australian - got me slightly drunk on Dutch gin and cut off my beard and trimmed my shoulder-length hair. I still didn't know who I was.

I remember, early on, going up to someone who'd lived in the place for a while and saying, "Excuse me... would you mind telling me what to do next?" He smiled enigmatically and said, "Sit. Just sit. Don't even read."

So that was what I did. There was an open verandah near my hot little room. Every day I'd go there after breakfast and sit. There was a whitewashed wall with scarlet bougainvillea growing across it. I'd sit there, sweating in the moist heat, and look at bougainvillea, feeling really weird. I was being deconstructed. My old self, my old patterns, were being disassembled and scoured.

One day I wrote a list of the names of all the women I'd made love to, and sat there by the white wall remembering them.... *Ann, Patricia, Betty, Carol, Geraldine, Shuri, Melonia, Danielle, Miranda, Barbara, Ruth, Tina...* I could feel them all in me, like ghosts. Not just memories. More... this is tricky so bear with me please... more like presences. They were still with me. There was so much to be thankful for - the love, the laughter, the closeness, the pleasure... But I could feel how sex had loaded their feelings into me, how full my being was of *their* energies.

I was going – I realized later - through a process of cleansing. Awakened by the Subud spiritual practice, there was a powerful force moving outwards through my various layers, shaking up or loosening whatever undesirable stuff it encountered and bringing it to the surface to release it through movement or words or sensation. I was being purified. Some of this process was extremely painful. At times I was feeling, all over the inside my skin, a multi-ant-bite sensation that was so intense I was scraping myself hard against walls and furniture to ease it, and lying face down on the floor murmuring through my drool: *"I'm sorry I'm sorry I'm sorry..... Please take this from me.... "*

Every night I went walking around in the soft tropical darkness muttering the same pattern of words over and over again: *"Dead end end ended deadened dead ended deadened end ended dead end.... "* Fortunately the locals were used to psychic refugees arriving from the West and behaving oddly.

I had no idea what was happening, but I trusted it. I felt like a kind of cipher, a non-entity. All I could do was maintain a basic survival program: eat at meal times, sleep when it was time to sleep, and sit for long silent hours by the red blossom glowing against the hot white wall. Little by little, as my inner was cleansed, I began to figure out what was going on. For the first time in my life I began to understand – no, *experience* - how they had affected me, the affairs I'd had and the drugs I'd taken.

As the teaching job came closer I began to feel relatively normal. It was as though the angels, or God, or whoever/whatever was running this cleansing process saw I was going to be around for a while, and that had I had a job to go to, and passed the word: "*Okay, we can ease up on him.*" Soon, as normal as I could be with my psyche in deconstruction mode, I was back in a classroom with a bunch of kids, they whom I love. I was okay, and I was going to be okay.

I lived in Cilandak for seven years. During that time I went through a brief, disastrous marriage and long periods of celibacy and solitude. It was a kind of purgatory. I was reconstructed. I became lighter and clearer in my being. I came to understand in my soul, in my guts, in my mind and my heart, in my toenails and in the lobes of my ears this truth: *sex harms me if I abuse it*. Finally, twice the man I ever was, I flew back to the West.

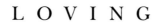

L O V I N G

How Having Sex Affects Us

The first letting in.
And then opening,
that's it, isn't it?
It's the opening so deep
that all the ancestors enter
& then you're tied forever
& even years later
like a quickening
you feel it,
like someone
whispering
inside you.
- Rasunah Katz

After my most intense cleansing phase I began to understood that the sexual relationships I'd had when I was a teenager and young adult had loaded me up inwardly with the energies of my partners. I only became aware that these energies were there because the process of being cleansed of them was so painful (especially the antbite sensation – I still wince when I think of that) and also because, as they left, I felt clearer and lighter and more and more ME. I remember shaving one morning and looking at myself in the mirror with a broad smile and saying, with an air of delighted discovery: "Oh, THAT'S who I am!" As the energies left in me by ex-lovers were dissipated I discerned a truth about sex that decades later I still believe. I'll repeat it: *Sex harms me if I abuse it.*

What I didn't know then was whether this truth was personal or general; true for me only, or true for other people as well, as in: *Sex harms us if we abuse it.* To answer this I needed to find out if there were others who'd undergone similar experiences and reached similar conclusions. Also, I wanted to understand *why* sex can be harmful... what's going on here? What was the nature of these energies from ex-lovers that I'd became aware of in my being? Thus began the search for answers of which this book is a part.

I met someone - Salamah Pope – with a similar story:

"I had always enjoyed the company of men. I had been fairly, but not wildly promiscuous... Now, ten years later, I realized that each and every one of those men had left his own distinct impression on, and in, me. I was full of 'foreign material.' How then could I be myself? As the process of spiritual purification went on, it had to disturb those long forgotten imprints, and bring them up to consciousness again, before they could be erased, and purified out of me..... I plunged into a period of total despair.... My agony was complete, my 'dark night of the soul' was on me....

It didn't disappear all at once, my darkness. In fact it took months for my depression to finally lift. But from that moment I knew that the core of the thing had finally gone, and that there was hope, again, in the distance...." –

Salamah arrived at conclusions very similar to mine: *"... with sexual activity, the influences from our partners are so strong that they go right through the layers around our own pure self, and imprint on it. So it's dangerous to one's own self to get involved in having casual sex. Our own pure feelings become contaminated, mixed up, by things and feelings from the other person, and lose their simple me-ness."*

This was so close to my experience and understanding that I knew there was a lot more than coincidence at work. Her words were enough to persuade me that "my" truth about sex might well be "our" human truth about sex. *When you have sex the energies that are alive and dominant in your partner enter your being and stay there.*

Why, I wondered, have I never encountered this truth before? Why isn't it part of our folklore, our culture, like "Money isn't everything" or "Elbows aren't the same as armpits"? We talk endlessly about sex without, apparently, arriving at this core truth. Maybe it's buried somewhere in the abstinence manifestoes or Tantric sex manuals. I discovered it only because, rather unusually, I spent a couple of decades as a serial monogamist in the West followed by seven years of spiritual purification on the island of Java.

Salamah went to live in Australia with her husband, and I came to California and got married. Years later she sent me a manuscript entitled "Sex and Sadness", which was her attempt to write a book about sex. Terrible title, I thought. "Emmanuel," she said, "I can't put it all together. YOU write the bloody thing."

This was about six years ago. I figured I'd understand a lot more about sex – and about life - if I wrote about it. Also, I thought a book about these aspects of sex I'd been thinking about might be useful to others. People like you for example. So I said okay.

I realized I needed other people to tell their stories about how sex can affect you, so I put the word out, and waited.

The first response was an email I received from a young Dutch woman:

Once I had sex with my boyfriend and afterwards I started very quietly to cry. I did not understand these tears. We have had fun! He had been very good to me, I was content and my body was really satisfied. I had nothing to complain about!

Still I felt the tears run down my cheeks and I felt a very very deep sadness.

It was not the first time this happened to me.

But it was the first time that someone asked me why I was crying, because other girlfriends of him had sometimes the same experience. And no one had ever given him an answer. He hoped I would.

My first reaction was to tell that it was for happiness.

Maybe because my mind could not find any reason to be sad.

To this man I said I did not really know.

I never really forgot this question, especially because I was not the only woman with this experience. It took me a long time before I was honest enough to admit that my soul was sad. My soul, I called it, as it was something deep down in my chest, behind my heart. That was something that I could not reason with...

Once I admitted that my soul was sad, although all the rest of me was happy, I felt I was right. And that my soul was very very much affected by sex. But I still do not understand really how.

Now I know that some men might be beautiful and really good men, but not the right person to have sex with. And another could be my right and true husband but the moment might not be right. But with the right person AND the right time ... No words for that.

There were lots more. Here's a selection:

Paul, married to Wendy for 30 years, told me about this experience:

4

It was just before we got married. I dreamt I was looking into a cave, standing at the entrance to it. The walls were wet. At the back of the cave there was a group of men. When they saw me they shouted and cheered and waved at me to come in and join them. I had no idea what was going on, but I felt like I shouldn't go into the cave.

Later I figured that the men in the cave were old lovers of Wendy. She'd gone through a phase of having sex with men because she was needy, she was looking for love. It was as though the dream was telling me about this and warning me that we would have some hard times to go through before our union would be clear.

There was no judgment, no blame in this. If anything, I felt more love for her.

Sometimes these traces, or energies, are dramatically apparent. An old friend sent me this account:

I was sleeping with an older Middle Eastern man. He really didn't want me other than for sex, whereas I pathetically pursued him.

One night, we had just had sex, and he was lying beside me sleeping. I woke up, and felt myself to be lying beside a rotten corpse. No, he wasn't dead, but later I realized that I was experiencing his inner condition. I was truly disgusted.

This experience made me stop sleeping around. Looking back, I see it's a pity that I had to keep it up until God gave me a truly ugly experience to make me stop. And I can tell you, that feeling of that experience did not go away. I still can feel it as I speak of it. I don't know if it has been purified out of me or not, but I'm sure I'd be better off without it.

When I came to live in California after my years in Java I got to know a funny, fast-talking, slightly nervous young woman – Andrea - who was physically obsessed by a man who had no feeling for her. He lived in an RV near a wood. In spite of herself, in spite of all her good intentions and resolutions, she'd drive over and knock at the door of his RV and plead with him to let her in. She wanted me to agree (I couldn't!) that he was handsome, and 'cool', and that he loved her, even though it was clear that he didn't. He had an enormous dog, I remember, that was always licking its private parts with a wet sloppy tongue.

One night she drove over there and the RV was gone. Empty space. That was it. No note, No phone call. Nothing. She sat in her car and cried for a long time.

Later she told me about a dream she had:

> *I cooked this beautiful meal.*
> *Everything was just right. Candles.*
> *White tablecloth.*
> *Silver cutlery all gleaming and everything*
> *and fine glasses for the wine.*
> *And the food had this feeling in it*
> *I mean it wasn't just that it tasted so delicious*
> *it had this quality in it*
> *because I felt so quiet and loving while I was*
> *cooking it.*
> *And then I carried the table out of the house*
> *and put it in the middle of the road*
> *and this huge great truck came roaring along*
> *and crushed it and smashed it all over the road.*

We've been friends for over thirty years. The RV man was her low point. She's fine now.

One young woman I know was living in a college dorm and for a while in her first year was having sex with a different guy pretty well every week. She was known as a slut, and was proud of it. Then she went home for Christmas. On the night of Christmas Eve she dreamt that she was giving birth, and when the babies came out of her body they had horns sticking out of their heads, and instead of crying they made weird hissing sounds. She was giving birth to demons. She figured the dream was a kind of warning, and when she returned to college after the holidays she went celibate.

Here's another story, from a young man named Miguel:

We lay there in the night's stillness, naked on the new beige carpet covering the living room of our Victorian house. Excitement coursed through our bodies and our hearts beat rapidly, endorphins enhanced by the illicitness of our union. She was still going out with my best friend, asleep in his bed two floors above. Though their relationship was ending, and though she and I loved one another, this was still his girlfriend. And knowing he or anyone could find us there made us all the more aware.

Side by side we lay and talked and kissed, slowly getting to know each other, patiently praying that we would do what we were doing in a good way, with awareness. Then I saw them. I looked on her face and saw beings inside her wanting to get out. Instead of her soft features, I saw men, clear faces from past affairs glowing red and green inside her. Then I saw her face again, but now she looked dark and ugly, a tainted spirit calling for rescue, calling for help suppressing the anguished voices inside.

I'm not kidding. This was not some trick of the light or an orgasmic hallucination. This was not due to any drink or drugs. I still remember the experience clearly...

Then more: she saw a ghost or spirit hovering above our heads, just watching with interest. I chased the spirit away with a flurry of angry phrases, but I could not chase away the spirits inside her. Sex is powerful.

We ended our tryst soon after and neither of us has so much as kissed another in the two years since; two years plus of self-regulated celibacy because of what we experienced in this sexual situation. Sex is serious. It shows things that aren't always

7

visible. I saw the imprint left in her spirit from careless liaisons and unresolved partners. I saw enough to scare me celibate.

Quite a few girls and young women, hoping to preserve their purity, have oral sex with men. Here's Rossie's story:

After my marriage broke up I had the strong feeling to go celibate for a while. So I went without a man for a long time. It was ok. Actually, it was good.

Then last year I met a guy... there was this really strong buzz between us, a powerful physical attraction. I really wanted him. But I also wanted to hold back. I felt like I'd got myself together, and come closer to God, and I didn't want to lose this feeling.

In the end we did have a relationship. We had sex.

But I had this strong kind of warning in me not to lose myself in the relationship. I felt I had to protect myself.

So I only had oral sex with him. I thought this would make me less vulnerable.

It was very sexual, very passionate between us. But after a while I knew it wasn't right for me so I ended it.

After I stopped seeing him I started getting these intense pains in my vagina. I went to the doctor and had all sorts of tests done but physically there was nothing wrong with me.

I didn't know what to do. The pain was terrible. I kept asking: "What is this terrible pain? Why am I feeling this pain?"

I received - my inner received - an understanding about what was going on. I understood that every time the man I'd had this relationship with thought about me, I experienced this pain..

I was shocked to discover that oral sex had had such a powerful effect on me, and that my belief that not having intercourse with him would mean I'd be ok was wrong. I was kind of angry for a while. In a way. It didn't seem fair.

After about three months the pains tapered off.

I'm okay now.

Therapist Thomas Moore, in his book The Soul of Sex, says that the physical uncovering of oneself in sex is mirrored by the soul's emergence from its protective covering. And he describes clients who complain that when they're having sex with their partner they suddenly and unexpectedly find themselves visited by fantasies of their partner's ex-lovers.[1]

I had an experience similar to this:

While I was living in London I met a woman called Elizabeth She was a new teacher at my school. We got to know each other, were attracted, dated.

A strange thing happened the first time we made love.

I saw in my 'mind's eye' a thickset, balding, bearded man in his early thirties. He was playing the saxophone. I even knew his name. Chuck. Later, I asked her who Chuck was.

"What?" she mumbled sleepily.

"Chuck. Who is he?"

"Why do you ask?"

"Plays the sax does he?"

By this time she was wide awake, sitting up in bed staring at me. I described the image I had seen. I said he had a dominating, manipulative feeling about him. After a while she told me about her affair with Chuck. It had ended about six months before she met me.

Here's a very approximate explanation of this experience:

Elizabeth had had a relationship with Chuck. When she slept with him she took in his energies. Then the relationship ended. Later she met me, and our intimacy reawakened the Chuck-energies still present in her inner. I wasn't sure - and I'm still not sure - exactly what these energies are, but I think they're there even if we don't feel them. In fact, because they're so close to us and so subtle we probably don't feel them.

Not all the stories were dark. Here's one man's account of three quite different experiences:

Years ago I made love to my wife and it was very pleasurable. Later I realized that when we made love I had been in the wrong state. We made love again and my penis became a sword and she had a miscarriage.

The night we conceived our second son we were making love and suddenly we were way up high in the sky. I could look down and see the earth. Now I understand those painting by Marc Chagall of lovers levitating.

The night our third son was conceived I felt a bolt or ray of energy, like electricity, shoot down from above through the top of my head, down my spine and into my penis. Straightaway I went upstairs to my wife. He's an unusual boy. Everyone he meets he touches their feelings.

An Indonesian man recorded this about making love with his wife:

"All about us, everywhere we looked, we saw various kinds of flowers which gave a very fragrant smell, and the stars seemed to be very close to us."

An old friend told me this story:

It was in 1974. I met this man. My marriage was over. He was married, but estranged from his wife. I had a very strong feeling I should be with him. Also, I felt that if we made love, for me, it would be like being crucified. We were going to get together, but I knew my period was due. I walked around a park on the edge of the city and had my entire period in two hours. We didn't make love... just held one another. A whole realm of things happened.

He went off with another woman. Left his family for her. This was in 1974. He'd call me from time to time, over the years. He always asked me to forgive him.

He called again a year and a half ago. This was after over thirty years. I'd been celibate all that time. We had dinner. We said we'd be entirely honest with one another. Our conversations have the effect of reminding ourselves of who we are, and of keeping one another on the right path. I'm not even attracted to him, physically. There's a deep love and tenderness.

When we made love we felt waves of light passing through us. Both of us felt that. We had a complete understanding of one another. We felt the power of our human souls connected to the power of God. It was a gift from God. We're joined. I've never experienced anything like this before. It's beyond the personal, beyond the understanding of our minds.

An English writer told me:

We'd been working for months to arrange the bar-mitzvah of our eldest son. My wife Rebecca and I decided to hold the ceremony in our bedroom. It just felt like the right place. It was a big, beautiful room that could accommodate all the guests.

Finally the big day came, and it was great! Everything went well, and the ceremony was truly a profound experience for all of us. That night, after it was all over and we'd cleared everything away, Rebecca and I made love. And there were so many angels in the room as we united I didn't think I'd be able to move. The place was packed.

(I read recently that the French call making love: "Voir les anges – to see angels".)

Stories are about what we experience. Ideas are what we put together with our minds when we want to understand what we experience. I've been asking myself: How do I make sense of the stories people sent me? What idea is big enough to contain the dark and the light of them? A woman sees the inner state of the man she has just had sex with as that of a "rotten corpse." A couple making love discover that they're miles about the earth; another couple that their room is full of angels. Sex will take us to heaven or to hell. Or, if you prefer, it will lift us up to unimaginable heights or drag us down to unimaginable depths. If this is true – and it's what I conclude when I read these stories and look for some simple, unintellectualized summary - then there's something to be understood here, which is:

Sex is never casual.
It is powerful.
It is not to be played around with.

You are, of course, free to respond to what I'm saying with doubt and skepticism.

"Where's your proof Emmanuel?"

"I don't have any."

"How much research have you done?"

"Well, I read a lot of books (over 100) but they don't talk about this. So they weren't much help. Plus I talked with a lot of people. Collected stories."

"Yes… these stories… do you have any evidence that they're true?"

"Do you mean, did the man making love with his wife take a photograph to prove that they were miles above the earth? Or the young man kissing the girl… did he whip out a camcorder and film the " *men, clear faces from past affairs, glowing red and green inside her…*"?

"Well…"

"No. I have evidence but no proof. You are, of course, free to dismiss everything that I, and a number of other people, are saying."

So what are they, these energies I've been talking about? I could sidestep the question and simply claim that however casually we treat it, *sex is a spiritual act,* and since the spiritual realm is beyond words there's nothing more to be said. However, over the past few decades scientists have been exploring phenomena that seem relevant to this enquiry. One way of acquiring some understanding of the energies involved in having sex is to consider what have been called 'fields'.

FIELDS

The basic substructure of the universe is a sea of quantum fields....
          – Lynn MacTaggart

The room you're sitting in is full of waves of energy, or fields. There's the gravitational field, without which you'd be floating around the room. There are transmissions from thousands of radio and television stations, some close, others thousands of miles away. There may be waves emitted by your computer and by your cell phone. There are light waves, sound waves, smell waves, and waves of energy radiating out from you.

Fields can pass through one another. They interpenetrate. They can occupy the same space in ways that bodies, stones, tree trunks and houses cannot. Think of a large hall full of people. Think of all those weighty visible physical presences with names and skin, clothes, blood, feet and bank accounts... and think of all those unseen energies radiating outwards from each person, auras maybe, like the glowing fields of energy around living entities captured in Kirlian photography, fine as music or aromas, passing back and forth through one another. Every human gathering is a jamboree of waves passing through one another, a chorale of unseen interpenetrationings. We may not be conscious of them, but if these radiating energies suddenly departed we'd feel painfully bereft. [1]

I want to take this wave idea and apply it to our central theme. Let's take it step by step:

* If we can accept the existence of subtle energies moving outwards from us, passing through subtle energies that are moving towards us from others …
* and if we can accept the idea that these energies have their center within us and that this center is the soul, or the inner, or essence, or whatever we want to call it…
* then we may be able to accept the possibility that having sex with someone is not just a physical joining of body to body accompanied by loud breathing and accelerating rhythms, but an exchange or interpenetrating of subtle energies …
* and that these energies may remain in our inners after the sex is over; linger still in her days later as she takes notes in a college lecture room, in him as he sits at a computer working on a website.

Currently, this is as close as I can get to understanding the energies exchanged in sexual intercourse.

Females, I believe, are more open to this imprinting process, because in love-making the female, however aggressive she may be, is essentially the *receiver* of energies, and the male is the transmitter, the source. An English friend says this: *"It's not a question of morals, as we observe that different cultures have varying practices. It's more*

to do with consequences. There is the possibility of real damage,
especially for the woman who, like it or not, is the vessel or
recipient. Who do you mix yourself up with?"

This gender difference may explain why traditionally
we've been much more protective towards unmarried
girls than unmarried boys, a protectiveness often
translated into a highly chauvinistic double standard
expressed by the terms 'stud' and 'slut' or 'hoe'. My
experiences in Indonesia, however, convince me that
males are also deeply affected by lovemaking. Yes,
women are the receivers and men the transmitters....
but it's always true that intercourse involves an *exchange*
of energies.

These energies are never neutral. They're not like
the taste of a peanut butter sandwich. They're not like
water running over a rock, or the wind pushing at clouds.
Some energies are higher, some are lower. Their quality
is determined partly by the level of being of each of the
sexual partners and partly by how they're feeling at the
time, by the nature of the act. Content and context. If
it's sex that's paid for – in prostitution or in porn - then
the energies will be low. If the partners have just had
a fight and are still angry but are having sex anyway,
the energies will be low. If she's too drunk to know or
care what's going on and he's after nothing more than a
quick screw, then the energies will be low. If the partners
are deeply committed to one another and pray before
they come together and are tender in their loving, then
the energies exchanged will be high.

I can't PROVE any of this. Certainly the stories
quoted in the previous section point in this direction.
As I said, try to feel out what I'm saying in your guts, in
your intuition.

If we think back to the room full of people, then
this question may arise: why aren't they vulnerable to

the energies moving in and out and all around them in the way that people having sex are? Seems like a daft question, I know, but let's have a look at it.

The people in the room are, let's say, fairly relaxed. But they are all wearing their social, or professional, identities, so there are layers around their souls. They're not vulnerable. When we take our clothes off to be naked with one another, we may put aside not only our clothes but our personas. And at the moment of orgasm, the soul or essence sheds its protective shield and is exposed and vulnerable. I think sexual intercourse opens us to a degree unmatched by any other human activity. This is why it has the capacity to lift us so high or drag us so low.

I suggest very speculatively that the main carrier of these energies between partners who are having sex is bodily fluids. Intimate sex, be it oral, anal or genital, involves an exchange of fluids. Water, as we are discovering, acts as a tape-recorder, one that not only sends the signal but amplifies it.

Here's another idea to ponder: If, not long ago, (say over the last two years or so) your partner had sex with a number of other people, *then he/she still carries the energies of these past lovers, and when you have sex, these energies will enter you.*

Think back to the Thomas Moore quote about clients who complain that when they're having sex with their partner they're "*suddenly flooded with fantasies of former lovers of their partner.*" I'm suggesting that these aren't fantasies they're flooded with, it's ghosts. Imprints. Energies from partners – old or current - that are still alive in the inner. It doesn't make sense to me that a woman having sex would fantasize (presumably sexually) about her partner's old girlfriends.

If this is true, then the convention that the sexually experienced man or woman is likely to be a better lover may be valid on the technical or even psychological levels. But spiritually, or on this subtle level, the reality is probably very different.

Here's something else to think about. I suggest – on the basis of experience - that we all have a 'voice' inside us. It's the voice of our inner, or our soul. It's the instrument that God, or the great life force, uses to warn or encourage us, so it's our source of guidance. However, if we sleep around, other people's energies enter and encumber us, making it harder it is for us to hear our inner voice. Imagine people in times of war, listening to the radio, trying to hear news of how things are going…. but there's heavy interference from storms, and maybe the broadcast is being jammed, and the people grouped around the radio can't hear what they need and want to hear because there's too much static.

Right when we have a more urgent need for guidance it's harder to access it.

Not all is lost when this happens. It's never true to say – and much comfort have I drawn from this - that all is lost. God – or the great life force, or the universe - is always trying to get through to help us. There I was living in a hippie house, hurt by a broken relationship, and an old friend sent me a telegram which introduced me to a bunch of kids who knocked the crap out of me and cleared enough space in me for my voice to get through and tell me that I was on a downhill path and needed to make some major changes, and I boarded a plane and flew to Indonesia.

Sitting for a long time by that hot white wall, looking at scarlet bougainvillea and feeling the energies of old lovers being moved around within me, I realized that these energies weren't all the same. What *she* left in me was different to what *she* left in me. Some of these energies were higher than others. So there's another aspect of this exchange-of-energies-in-lovemaking subject that I want to explore.

Basic Levels of Being

Your level of being attracts your life

— Gurdjieff

During the white wall days I would observe how my feelings were affected by memories. I'd suddenly shake my head and realize I'd been completely lost for, well, I didn't know how long, lost in a time other than now, a year or a decade ago, my body and heart re-experiencing the up or the down feelings of back then. Little by little, day by day, I got better at watching this happen. I was becoming a more vigilant observer of my inner life, and, as a result, was no longer totally immersed in or swayed by these roller-coaster feelings. Slowly there emerged a deeper, quieter me who was beginning to understand how I had always been helplessly pulled up, down and about by my experience of the world. "*Maybe,*" I thought, "*I can become a better person.*" Peering uncertainly at this future me I found myself hoping I wouldn't be boring. It can sometimes seem that our faults are what make us interesting.

There were radiant memories and dark memories, and when I considered them I saw that every experience affects me in some way. I remember sitting there in the hot afternoon shade saying solemnly to myself: *There are no neutral experiences.* Everything I take in or participate in, I realized, be it horror films or romantic comedies, casual sex or deeply loving union, either affirms or denies me, raises me up or pulls me down.

As a primrose path man I'd never had any sense of a scale or hierarchy in which things I do, influences I am subjected to, energies that enter my being can be placed in higher or lower categories according to their content. But I was seeing that the energies or traces left in me by the women I'd been involved with were different, not just in the ways that we're all different, or unique, but different in ways that I had to identify as "higher" or "lower". My primrose path guideline, if I'd had one, could have been summed up as: *If it feels nice it's okay,* with a dash of *If I can still make a fool of myself over a woman, I'm still alive.*

I remembered a teacher at a school I was working at. Olivia. She came to my classroom one afternoon after the kids had had gone home. Wanted some ideas on how to make math more interesting for her 4th graders. She was slow in her speech and ways, slow and thoughtful. Unusually, if she didn't have anything to say she said nothing. I set her up with some math games I'd evolved. She invited me to dinner a few nights later. We didn't make love; we just had a sweet, gentle romp, which led to me prancing around her studio room laughing with joy. Next day, I remember, we were all gathered in the hall for morning assembly. The principal announced the hymn: "*Lord we thank thee for this night,*" and Olivia and I exchanged secret smiles.

When, sitting by the white wall, I thought of Olivia, I felt the laughter again and the lightness, and I wondered why the memory of her should make me feel so euphoric. I remembered another girl, Miranda, with whom I'd been involved. She and her house-mates threw a big party, and I found her making out with someone else, and walked out. Months later she rang me, said she wanted to go for a picnic in the country. She lay in the grass and reached out for me. I said, "Do you know what you're doing?" and she said "Yes." Afterwards, as we walked back to the car there was a heavy downward silence between us, as though gravity had grown stronger.

I'm not sure whether it's the quality of one's partner that may be high or low, or the quality of the love-making. I think it can be either, or both. But I was figuring out, on those long hot days by the white wall, that we're not all on the same level, or, to put it another way, we're not all at the same point on our journeys. There were girls who really had pulled me down. I'd been a willing partner in our downward dance, so I'm not judging them. And there were one or two who had – so it felt – enveloped me in radiance.

I was thinking that maybe people have different levels of being. Let's bring this idea to life in a scenario:

Here's 20 year-old Maggie, good at sports, loves kids, studying to be a music therapist, has an open, generous heart. Maggie's in love with a 24 year-old who goes by the name of Steelhead. Steelhead's a doper who's trying to quit. He thinks Maggie's totally cool. In fact, he can't quite work out what it is she sees in him. Neither can any of her or his friends. Steelhead's a dj. Not a particularly successful one, because he doesn't really push himself to succeed at anything.

Maggie thinks he has real talent as a musician. He played her some songs he composed when he was in his teens. She thought they were great, and she's always encouraging him to write more, or do a good demo of some of his stuff, but he never quite gets round to it. He tends to make promises - to himself and others - that he doesn't keep.

Maggie gets angry when he gets stoned. He reacts to her irritation, and they have a fight, and stop seeing each other for a few days. Steelhead's always the one who does the calling up, who says sorry, who promises it won't happen again.

Although he may not have worked it out very clearly, Steelhead sees Maggie as someone who can help him get his act together, who can 'save' him. He also likes the idea of having sex with a cheerleader type. She's quite different to any girl he's been out with before. Sometimes he genuinely tries to live up to her belief in him, and get his act together. He's a slightly better person because of her. He's been faithful to her, for example, which for him is a first.

And Maggie? Well, she's attracted by Steelhead's street smarts, by his sexuality, by his slightly 'beat-up' club charisma. Maybe part of her is reacting to the fact that she's always been a model student who worked hard and got high grades. She enjoys his easy-going style, his cheerful irresponsibility, even as she's dismayed by it. And she loves him.

If the relationship continues, Maggie may lose a lot of her idealism and generosity of heart. She's already less clear and light in her feeling, although she's not aware of it. She's getting cynical, and there are days when she feels down for no reason. She can't 'save' Steelhead. Only he can do that, and he's probably going to need a real shock of some kind before he does.

Maggie's lamp, we could say, is clear and bright because the oil of her essence is clean. Steelhead's oil is quite thick and dirty, but the light his being gives out is colorful because he has tinted glass in his lamp. This disguises the quality of his inner. Maggie is taken in by this. And because she's in love with him, she doesn't try to see any further than the colors.

So here's what I've worked out from my early understandings by the white wall, and over the years since then. I call it the B.L.O.B. theory.

Basic Level of Being - B.L.O.B. - has nothing to do with class, ethnicity, culture or religion or anything like that. It has to do with the qualities, or energies, alive and dominant in someone's inner, and I'm suggesting that these qualities may be high, fine or light; or low, coarse or dark. Say you're involved with someone who's pressuring you to do drugs, or weird sex, or who's drinking a lot, or hurting or betraying you, then that person's basic level of being may be lower than yours, especially if you don't feel comfortable or okay about what they're trying to get you to do. However much you love that person, their level of being is not going to change quickly, and you might want to think hard about whether this person is right for you. Remember: *your first responsibility is to yourself.*

On the other hand, your partner may be someone you find yourself trusting, without even thinking about it. Somehow you know that he or she isn't going to let you down, isn't going to hurt you, or, if they do, it was unintentional and they acknowledge what they did and ask your forgiveness. And you laugh a lot together, and sometimes know what each of you is thinking before it's said. They bring out the best in you. Loving them you love yourself. Even if you're not in such a relationship, if you can feel the quality of such love, feel what it's like, then you may recognize this as what you want, and give yourself to nothing less.

(If you want a clearer understanding of what is meant by "higher" and "lower" qualities, you might jump out of sequence here and read through the "Life Energies" section in the appendix.)

We affect and are affected by one another all the time. When you think obsessively about someone, you attract that person's energies into your being. If you're totally in love with someone and can't stop thinking about him/her, then your psyche takes in that person's energies, or qualities, whether you're actually with them or not. You may have noticed, for example, how sometimes you hear yourself talking just like one of your friends, using their favorite expressions.... Even *sounding* a bit like them...

So, when you do your list of 'my ideal guy', 'my ideal girl' (and most of us do when we're young) remember the BLOB factor. It will help you find someone with a level of being that's roughly the same as your own. This isn't easy though, because *who we really are is invisible.*

Let's look at invisibility.

Invisible People

We do not grasp that we are invisible. We do not realize that we are in a world of invisible people. We do not grasp that life, before all other definitions of it, is a drama of the visible and the invisible.

- Maurice Nicoll

Pondering by the white wall on my primrose path days, I saw that most of my ex-lovers were physically beautiful and that the ones who hurt me the most tended to be the most attractive. Beauty, I realized, has nothing to do with what the person's like inside. We all know this, but it's worth re-stating. Physical beauty has nothing to do with who a person is *inwardly*. Who we really are can't be seen, because *we are invisible people*.

If we're hung up on the physical we may turn away from someone who would have been a wonderful partner for us just because she has a big butt or he has acne. Our thoughts, feelings, dreams, fantasies, memories, hopes, fears, ambitions, talents, worries, desires, regrets, beliefs, likes and dislikes… all these make up who we really are, and they are mostly invisible. As is our soul.

We may often feel that we are invisible, that other people seem to know nothing of who we are, of what we are feeling, of our deep need for love and acceptance. But we don't really grasp that others are just as invisible to us. Although we've learnt a lot about our inner lives over the last century or so, we still live in a world of invisible people, one reason being that our culture places so much emphasis on physical appearance that we're conditioned to think that this is what's most important.

When I was a kid I used to bike to a stream that ran through the English countryside and explore it. There were little creatures called caddis grubs, who used whatever was around - bits of twig and weed stalk and tiny stones - as material that they glued together to make tunnels that they lived inside. I think we do this as we grow towards adulthood – we use whatever's around in our community and culture to construct personalities, or egos, that we live inside. Unlike caddis grubs we can change the look of our tunnels. We can develop different personalities - who we are when we're with our friends, with our boy/girlfriend, with a supervisor, teacher, parent, little sister or brother. We may act sophisticated and sexy, we may play at being the macho guy, we may play the lone wolf (an old one of mine), the outsider, the clown, the heavy drinker, the Goth, the stud, the druggie, the nerd, the jock, the intellectual, the party girl, the slut, the rebel, the geek, the fashion model, the dude, the streetwise guy. And, beneath these selves, behind these images, there's this new psyche forming…. the embryo, we might say, of our adult identity.

There will always be parts of us that remain invisible, even to ourselves (there are as many inner as there are outer dimensions), but the more visible we can safely be with someone the closer we are to our true selves. So we may remind ourselves that this person we're attracted to is mostly invisible, and that it'll take a while before we get to know what the invisible he or she is like so maybe we should wait a while before coming too close.

In loving union, there is trust, so there are no secrets. Nothing is held back. Two invisible worlds are accessible to one another, with no frontiers, no border guards. Fields of fine energy flow into one another:

Let me see you.
Let me touch and be inside you.
Let me open myself to you as I have never done.
I will be all yours, all for you in a way
you have never experienced before.
I will flow beside you like water
and pillow you like the softest air.
A warm wind will be my breath,
and my hands will move upon you in
ways you have never known.
As the doorways into our bodies open,
we let each other inside, slowly at first, so that
we can feel every contour, the texture and size;
the softness, the exquisite softness,
knowing for certain there is nothing finer, richer,
or more exceptional than this that has ever existed,
or will ever exist again.
I'm waiting for you now.
I'm looking at you with shining eyes.
All you need do is glance in my direction,
      and neither of us turn away.
        - Paul Strom

Casual sex is body to body and ego to ego. The real he or she is invisible to you. Here are your bodies, as close as they can be, skin to skin, mouth to mouth, breath mingling with breath and sweat with sweat.... and there are your psyches, your real feelings, completely separate. Universes apart.

One reason why we get so caught up with how sexy someone *looks* has to do with "Sex in the Head." Instead of celebrating sex (perhaps the greatest gift for our earthly lives) our culture exploits it, enclosing us – through TV, magazines, internet etc. - in an environment of hyper-sexualized imagery, a "Pornotopia" as our sexualized culture has been called. As a result – for men in particular - our sexual energy moves from its rightful place in our bodies, into our heads. But the head, the mind, is too small a home for it, and our sexuality, with all its potential for passion and love, tenderness and transcendence, is reduced to the addictive cycle of stimulus, tension and release. Let's look more closely at this idea.

Sex In The Head

As a man, I would advise that we avoid sexual imagination: the danger of wrong use of the head.
                                              - Ronald Leask.

In Indonesia I knew an Armenian called Joe. Joe's life had been full of suffering. He lost his wife and kids in one war, and his parents in another. Joe showed me that people can go through several versions of hell and still smile.

I'd just returned after a summer vacation back in England. I'd been telling Joe about walking through central London, checking out the girls in their mini-skirts, the sex pheromones crackling across the streets like electricity. He nodded. "*Yah, yah …. the trouble with westerners, they got sex in the head. Sex belongs down there,*" he said, pointing to his guts. "*Most westerners, their sex is up here,*" pointing to his head.

It took me a while to understand what he meant by this remark. I could gain a clearer perspective on it back in Indonesia because the feeling between men and women in the streets and markets was a lot quieter… there's not the same hot automatic male - and female! - scanning of bodies characteristic of the West. Also, the culture – TV, music, advertising etc. - was a lot less sexually charged.

I remember a big Australian surfer I met in Jakarta called Mick. The story he told me illustrates how it is when the deeper sexual feelings are alive, even in a non-physical context:

Mick spoke Indonesian fluently. He was courting a beautiful Indonesian girl named Sri.

Sri's parents were quite traditional in their attitudes and morality. Sri could sit with Mick at a table on the patio outside her house. The maid would bring tea or coffee and Indonesian sweets. The parents would be in the house; neighbors would be passing by or visiting. It was a typical 'kampong', or village, situation, in which the almost total lack of privacy meant that everyone knew what everyone else was up to.

Mick would sit there opposite this lovely Javanese girl and sip tea and smile and make conversation. Sri's skin was a soft café-au-lait; her hair was thickly black and glossy, and her dark brown eyes had a kind of smoldering in their depths. Mick would have fantasies of driving away with Sri on the back of his motor- bike, off to some distant place where they could be alone.

Then there was the day Mick was sitting there, sipping his tea and looking across the table into Sri's eyes. She smiled at him. Neither of them said anything. Their gazes held each other. Then Mick felt a stirring deep in his guts, the like of which he'd never felt before. He kept looking into Sri's eyes, and, as he told me later, felt her sexual energy, deep and strong, moving across the space between them and embracing his body in warm waves. "Bliss", he said. "It was bliss."

His sexual energies were stirring and responding to hers.

"So we're sitting there," he said, "sitting at the table, with our tea and our coconut cookies, and it feels like we're making love. Blimey, mate."

Our culture is invisible to us until we step outside it. Returning to London after two years in Indonesia I saw how sexualized Western mass culture was. This was true even back in the mid-seventies, well before pornography became mainstream. Arriving in London at the end of a plane trip from Java was to experience, not culture shock – I was, after all, coming home – but spirit shock. We don't realize how blatant our popular culture has become. Many immigrants coming to the West from more traditional societies experience this spirit shock. The sex and violence are crass and crude and continually in your face. Tattania Mananova, a Russian feminist, commenting on the difference between the West and Russia, observed, *"The pornography.... It's everywhere, even on billboards.... (it) is a different kind of assault. And it doesn't feel like freedom to me."*[1]

The hyper-sexual images aimed at us in commercials, movies, magazines and the internet gradually push the sexual energy – particularly among men – out of its true home in our sex organs and into our heads. Virtuality and fantasy take over from real sex between real people who fight and laugh and love one another. A magazine picture of a moist-lipped woman in a bikini or of a tight-jeaned hunk is nothing more than tiny dots of color on paper, probably with boobs or abs digitally rearranged. We've been surrounded by so many of these images for so long they've become normal. Step back for a moment, though, and think about this. Isn't it strange that these mass-produced, one-dimensional, digitally manipulated, pixellated images arouse so many people? What would an E.T make of it?

"What this?" asks E.T.
"It's a picture of a sexy woman," says Steve.
"You like picture?"

"Yeah! It's sexy!"
"Is picture sexy?"
"Yeah! I mean like check out those boobs man!"
"How can picture be sexy? Can Steve mate with picture?"
"I can pretend I'm mating with her."
"Steve look at picture and pretend he mate with woman?"
"Yeah."
"But she not woman, she picture."
"Yeah well it's…"
"And she not your mate?"
"No."
"E.T. no understand."
"It's what we do here man…It's kind of hard to explain."

If oldies like me harrumph about the increasing sexualization of our culture and declining moral standards among young people then we'll probably be regarded as uptight puritanical killjoys. But I'm not talking here about declining moral standards among young people because I don't see them as declining. Fewer teenagers and college students are having sex. A 2006 survey found that nearly half of Harvard undergraduates reported that they had never had intercourse. As is often the case, the picture the media presents us of who we are and what we're doing is largely inaccurate. MTV porn, Girls Gone Bad, Desperate Housewives, no-underwear-Britney etc… this isn't how most of us live. As Stephanie Koontz observed: *"There's a lot more sex on television that there is in the bedroom."* [2]

Let me be clear about this: I'm not against sex. I'm against the increasingly blatant sexual content of our culture because I'm *pro-sex*. The soft porn imagery bombarding us daily has as much to do with real sex as violent video games have to do with real human pain and suffering. It dilutes and degrades our sexuality, pushing it out of its home in our sex organs and into the head.

Males – being primarily visually oriented - are particularly affected by sexual imagery. In our "Pornotopian" world there are boobs everywhere: plump boobs high boobs white boobs brown boobs firm boobs soft boobs tattooed boobs real boobs gel boobs filmed boobs videotaped boobs photographed boobs covered boobs semi-covered boobs and nude boobs. (One film critic memorably described the girls in a recent teen-targeted movie as: "*Life support systems for breasts*".)

As the author of Pornotopia observes:

Since pornography is the primary source of this imagery in our culture, it is hard to imagine what non-pornographic public representations of sexuality would even look like. The pornographic imperative is now so ubiquitous in language and imagery that it can hardly fail to influence the way in which young people think about their bodies, their desires and what they expect from their sex partners...[3]

Recently, in a supermarket, I had this insight: our hormones can't tell the difference between what's real and what's image. When eyes scan a Cosmo cleavage on a supermarket rack, hormones react as though it's a real woman smiling back, not an image composed of millions of tinted dots. But there's no one there, no living breathing human being with a vibrant inner world full of memories and secrets and longings; the scarlet smile stays fixed and the glossy eyes stare blankly at the cut-price avocados.

So then the hot surge, with nowhere to go, curls back in on itself and creates a fantasy, or gets pushed into a space that grows hotter and more crowded as the day passes. In Pornotopia this response (primarily male) to sexual imagery is constantly reactivated. Soon the organism is mildly addicted and tells the eyes to seek out more images for more arousal. The result is a build-up of sexual tension needing release, either through masturbation or sex with a partner. The latter probably won't last very long. Quick and shallow – ah that's better. After a while the images feeding this addictive force become too familiar. They don't do it any more. Something different is required to re-trigger the pleasurable stimulus, and we are drawn towards pornographic material that is progressively more extreme. Hundreds of thousands of people are being pulled into this addictive cycle, human beings losing their humanity to the drive to make money whatever it takes. In America the porn industry is worth about twelve billion dollars a year. I regard the easy accessibility and constant spread of porn with its inevitable consequence of more and more addicts as a very grave and urgent spiritual problem, a source of great and growing darkness in our human world.

Sexual union is what people do *together.* The more intimately together the couple is, the richer and more loving the union. Sex in the head is masturbatory and solitary. It's a closed loop. It doesn't need anyone else as a partner, as a complex human being with needs, likes, preferences of his/her own. All it wants is a body, or the image of a body. It wants virtual intimacy leading to an orgasm, to the sweet release of pressure, the honeyed numbness. Inevitably it leads to a darkening and lowering of the content of love-making.

Here's a married guy, let's call him Jack, looking at internet porn. He's watching sex that's performed for money. This is its purpose; this is its content. Money is a material force. It has no value in itself. Sex for money is material sex. So Jack is taking into his being material energy, which degrades his inner feeling. Jack probably thinks that doing porn has nothing to do with his marriage. He probably believes that it's a separate thing, a hobby like fishing or playing pool. A guy thing. However, it doesn't work like this. When he watches porn and masturbates it's not happening in some separate walled-off compartment inside him. Everything's connected. Jack's feelings for his wife are being degraded. If porn get Jack fixated on certain details - he wants her in *this* position or *these* clothes, or he wants her to get her boobs fixed or even her vagina because this is what his fantasies require, then – if she goes along with it - both partners are being used by a sub-human force intent on nothing but its own satisfaction. Their love-making is directed by his fantasies, which are in turn shaped and stirred by images *strangers made for money*.

"Surveying some of the survivors of wife assault," writes Susan G. Cole," I have encountered women who openly confess that their sex lives changed considerably once their husbands got into pornography. The pornography, often from magazines, gave their husbands all kinds of ideas about what was sexy… Many of these women reported being forced to replicate sexual acts in the pornography. …. In other words, pornography makes something happen in the bedroom." [4]

A friend who recently kicked his six-year porn addiction told me how porn had conditioned him to look at women as nothing but objects to be possessed with a teeth-clenched brutality.

Here's a true story told me by an old friend:

I had to go live in a hotel for a while. On the first night I felt that there was something on the bed. Next morning when I awoke I felt sexually excited, to the point that I could not control myself. I went to work and this feeling just kept getting stronger. After work I just wanted to be near a woman, any woman. That did not happen, but I wound up buying porn and masturbating.

This went on for three days. Finally, feeling very disturbed and desperate, I started to pray. As I prayed felt the presence of a large German Shepherd dog which was a lot stronger than I was. He was on top of me and had me pinned to the floor. I desperately called to God for help and received enough strength to get up and order the dog out of the room. Finally he left, and after a while I felt normal again.

Next evening I was back in the hotel room. I was thinking about porn, and the dog, and how I felt God had been helping me. Then I was made to lie on the floor and close my eyes, and this long stream of pornographic images started coming out of my body going straight up and disappearing in the air. It seemed like every sexual image that I had seen in my lifetime was being drawn out of me. When it was over, I felt a tremendous sense of relief and much cleaner inside.

Sometimes I wonder how it feels to be a girl or a woman, walking out in the world and being looked at and desired by men. An attractive woman once told me how wonderfully different she felt when she was obviously pregnant; for a while she was no longer the target of hungry male gazes. "Men look at women," says art critic John Berger. "Women watch themselves being looked at. This determines not only most relations between men and women but also the relationship of women to themselves. The surveyor of women in herself is male; the surveyed female. Thus she turns herself into an object – and most particularly a object of vision: a sight." [5]

I remember an English Composition class I taught in a Los Angeles college. There were about 15 students in it, mostly young men. We'd settled down well after a couple of sessions, and I was thinking we were going to have a friendly, productive semester together. Then a new student joined the class in the third session, and everything changed. She was a beautiful young woman, and she wore very revealing clothes and potent perfume. Nina.

So there was Nina, sitting in the class, and every student was affected one way or another by her presence. The other girls were uptight or competitive, and the guys were - subtly or crudely - competing for her attention. The atmosphere in the class deteriorated. I could see that she was aware of the effect she was having, and was thoroughly enjoying it. So one day I spoke to her after the class. I told her I had no wish to criticize her or hurt her feelings... but that she was having an unsettling effect on the class because she was attractive, and because she wore clothes that made her look very alluring and seductive. Many of the guys were finding it hard to concentrate. I asked her if she understood what I was saying, and if she agreed. She nodded. She looked embarrassed and awkward, which was quite natural. Then I asked her if there was anything she thought she could do to make the situation better. She said, "Okay, Mr. Williams, you want me to look less sexy, right?"

"Yes please," I said.

I had no right to ask this of her. For all I knew, I was breaking the law, or interfering with her rights, in even bringing the subject up. But I felt I had to.

Next session she was dressed much more modestly. At first there was a sense of disappointment among the guys. But soon we - Nina included - were able to focus a lot more on English Composition, which was, after all, what we were there for.

The male animal/human is programmed to ensure that survival of his species, so he seeks females with bodies that look sexually fertile. White teeth and glossy hair indicate youthfulness and good health. Full firm breasts and flaring hips suggest fertility. A slender waist indicates that the woman is not pregnant; therefore the male has no need to prove paternity.

So the animal instinct towards procreation and the survival of the species is part of our sexuality. However, there's a major difference between us and animals. If a baboon is aroused it will go ahead and mate, or try to. Since this is how it's biologically conditioned, it has no choice in the matter. But we humans can be sexually aroused... *and choose not to act on it.*

If we - men particularly - always followed the animal forces in our natures we might be killing the babies sired by the previous dominant male, or eagerly sniffing at one another's sex organs. Our biological conditioning would leave us no choice. But as humans we have the capacity to choose. And the more consciously we choose what we do, the more human we become.

Without choice we have no freedom.

The more choice we have, the more freedom we have.

This is why addictions are such a human tragedy. To become an addict is to lose much of the fullness of choice that our human potential urges us towards. Addictions are the logical outcome of a capitalist system dominated by the profit motive. *Whether they're addicted to pornography, alcohol, gambling, shopping, cigarettes or drugs, addicts are the ideal consumers.*

Except, of course, that many die before their time.

(For a brilliant analysis of consumer addictiveness see Benjamin R. Barber's book "Consumed" pp. 235 –249.)

Whoooooooo.
Heavy stuff. Take a deep breath. Have a glass of water.

And now for something completely different.

Take a moment to remember a time when you went camping in a forest or up in the mountains or by a lake ... Remember how everything was simpler and cleaner? Nobody was trying to sell you anything, or nag at your mind with STUFF, or turn you on with sexual imagery. Imagine for a moment how it would be if, in response to an enormous public outcry, our culture were cleaned of much of its pornographic content. Imagine: there are no television shows, no commercials or movies or magazines or internet sites or fashion billboards or songs or MTV videos *with heavy sexual content.* We'd be the inhabitants of Unpornotopia, a country in which there's much less virtual, commercialized sex directed at us by those who make so much money from it.

This isn't a total fantasy; in some ways it's the world I grew up in, and that millions of people still inhabit. If it exists it is possible.

How would it feel? How would it be different?

Sex wouldn't disappear, would it? Men and women would still flirt, and fall in love, and make love, and betray one another and hurt one another and delight one another.... there'd still be rape and babies, orgasms and abortions, weddings and divorces. But, ah, the changes we would have brought about.

Men wouldn't be going around feeling vaguely horny all the time. *Gee guys there are other things to think about.*

The human temperature would drop.

Children would stay innocent – which is what they should be - for as long as they are children.

Our sexuality would mellow and deepen. Human beings would desire real human beings, men or women they had feelings about, men or women with pasts and memories and dreams and fears and favorite movies and brothers and sisters and moms and dads and friends and stale breath in the morning, not computerized Simones on magazine covers, not jiggling singers; not this anonymous blonde with ropes scoring her skin hiding her pain and trying to look as though what these men are doing to her is just what she wants or at least just what she deserves.

I'm absolutely certain there'd be less rape. It is surely no coincidence that since porn entered American mainstream culture - beginning in the early sixties in magazines like Playboy and Penthouse, then moving into video and then on to the internet - the incidence of rape in U.S.A. has increased by approximately 500%.

I repeat: I'm speaking *in favor of sex.* I'm visualizing a world in which the insistent, sexual stimulus to which we are subjected by the media is turned way down, so that human passion and human love, with all its myths, promises and secrets, may grow.

All together now…

Turn it down
Turn it down
turn it down
turn it down

turn it down

turn it down

turn it down

Thank you

Visualize with me a world in which when we look at one another we see human beings, not shapes we measure up against some unreal sexual image planted in the space behind our eyes. A world in which our sexuality is stronger and deeper, *because it is ours.* Just as a spontaneous surge of joy, of leaping-about-in-the-sunlit-meadows-of-tingleforce is ours, fully and gloriously ours, when it's not the expression of a drug.

Obviously it's not my place to tell you to stop watching porn. I just want you to be able to make clearer choices about what you take in. You're the keeper of the gate that opens to your inner being. What passes through those gates is your responsibility. No one but you knows everything that you do in your life. Other people know some of it - your parents, your partner, your friends. But you're the only one who knows your habits, your secrets, your struggles and your dreams. You're the only one who can know your invisible world, your unseen self. It's important that you become familiar with your nature and with the impulses or forces that influence it. You have a big responsibility to yourself, and this includes working out what's right for you, and what isn't. Porn isn't. Porn isn't right for you. I wish I could stand before you and put my hands on your shoulders and look you in the eye and take a deep breath and say it with all the certainty that I feel in my heart and my lungs, my feet and my colon and my soul…

Porn is bad for you.

You have to do the best for yourself.

We all do.

Sooner or later we have to become our own boss.

Being the Boss

A little kingdom I possess,
Where thoughts and feelings dwell;
And very hard the task I find
Of governing it well.

- Louisa May Alcott

In the "little kingdom" of our beings there's a ruler and there are servants. When the ruler is enthroned and in command, then the kingdom is at peace, with everyone busy at their allotted tasks. If the ruler resigns or pretends not to be the ruler, one of the servants will take over the seat of authority, and chaos will reign.

The servants don't really want to be the ruler. When they usurp the throne they bring the ruler down to their level. In some ways they enjoy this, but what they really want is for the ruler to *lift them up*. So they'll test the ruler out, but they'd rather he or she was in charge. They're a bit like students who test the teacher. They're actually happier if the teacher is able to maintain order because then they can get on with what they're there for.

As I sat day after purgatorial day by the white wall in Java with its adornments of scarlet bougainvillea and watched old games and identities being dismantled,

I was – I realize now - looking for an answer to the question: "Who am I?"

"*I am the ruler,*" I told myself. "*I am the boss.*"

Mind you, I didn't yet know who the ruler was. I could tell myself - *I am the one who's always there, beyond moods, trends and images* - but I was still a long way from living with this ruler fully present and in charge. I was certainly getting better, though, at recognizing the servants. The servant who presents the biggest challenge is the sexual drive. The rewards that may (no guarantees!) come our way if we are able to master our sexuality are beyond words. But it's hard work. Here's a scenario:

This is Steve, and this is Wendy. Steve doesn't much like Wendy, but she's bending down to pick a book up and he's peering down the front of her blouse and he feels a hot sting in his privates…

Wendy knows that Steve is looking at her boobs; she senses it even though she isn't looking at him. She doesn't like Steve much either, but she likes to get guys to look at her body that way. Grunting inwardly like a gorilla, Steve watches her walk away, then checks out Deirdre and Christina as they walk towards him. They're both wearing tight tee shirts and he can see their boobs bouncing.

Follow Steve through the afternoon and evening, checking out the girls in the school carpark and the street, checking out the girls on MTV. By early evening he'll have gazed at scores of inaccessible boobs, and he's roaring inwardly like a space rocket stuck in the gantry. If he meets his girlfriend Martine tonight he'll be hot for it. If Martine's not free he'll find someone else, or he'll masturbate.

Steve's on automatic. He's not aware of what he's doing, of what's happening to him. Yes, his behavior is, in an animal way, natural. But – and this is one of the major ideas in this book - learning to be truly human is learning to be *more than animal.* It's not that the animal force in us is bad. It's a valued servant that gives us our drive to procreate, our sense of family and of tribe, our survival instinct, and our will. It gives us much of our culture. But when it comes to sexuality – and aggression - our human responsibility is to hold these forces in place so that we can act on them consciously, rather than being pushed and pulled around by them.

What this is about is deciding to stop automatically following these impulses in ourselves so that we can begin to live as human beings. We men are always leering at attractive women, checking boobs, butts, legs, faces etc., but there's no way we'll ever even talk to the vast majority of them, even if we had the time to. I'm a happily married man; I've been faithful for well over 20 years, and I'm quite old, but I still find myself doing the T. and A. scan of young women behind the coffee bar counter or across the street... and then I think to myself, "*Emmanuel, come on! What's the point?*" I remember an old friend telling me, with much rueful laughter, how she got married and then, if she was out with her husband and she looked at another man she tripped over her feet. Her husband thought she had some kind of physical problem until she told him what was going on.

There was an interesting experiment begun at Stanford University in the 1960s:

The Marshmallow Test.

A group of 4 year-olds were told that if they waited until someone had completed an errand, they could have two marshmallows. If you can't wait, if you want marshmallow now, then you can. But you can only have one.

About two thirds of the kids were able to wait. They covered their eyes, they sang, played games, tried to sleep. The rest went straight for their marshmallow as soon as the adult left.

These same kids were followed up 12 - 14 years later. The interesting thing is that the ones who were able to control their impulses and wait turned out to be self-confident, more able to face difficulties, self-reliant, able to make their own decisions and follow them through.

The other kids, the third who couldn't wait, were more likely to be socially awkward, easily frustrated and discouraged; to be resentful if they didn't get what they wanted, and more likely to get into fights. They even got lower scores in SAT tests. [1]

I'm not a neurologist, but I was interested to learn that, according to current research, there's a part of our brain that's wired to work with us in making these choices. It's the orbitofrontal area of the prefrontal cortex - OFC for short. It's positioned just behind the eyes and between the emotional centers and the thinking brain. Because it's connected to what might be called the "lower" brain areas – the amygdala (source of many emotional responses) and the brain stem (reptilian source of reflexive responses) and including the senses and the data they're sending - and the cortex, or the "higher" thinking brain, the OFC seems to be that part that looks at all the incoming data and evaluates it, finds meaning of some kind, and comes up with a plan of action. It's a kind of control center. It enables us to sort through impressions, emotional reactions and impulses and orchestrate our responses. It balances – as in the Marshmallow Test - our short-term and long-term interests. It's extraordinarily flexible, it can carry out a wider variety of tasks than any other part of the brain, and *it is much larger in us humans than in other primates.* It might be called The Boss.[2]

Following your impulses without examining them - *I want this so I'll have it; I want to do that and I'll do it* - looks like freedom. It isn't though. The energies generating these impulses are free. But you - potential human being that you are - you're not free. Not really. The servants – which we could call the "lower energies" - are in charge. A lot of people are working very hard to persuade the two-marshmallow kids to follow their impulses and go for the one marshmallow that's there, right in front of them. The American advertising industry spends three hundred and thirty billion dollars a year – nearly a billion a day - doing just this.

When we are able to separate ourselves from our habits and patterns, and from the pressures of these lower energies, we open a space in ourselves for something else, something higher. As Salamah puts it: *occasionally we do have flashes of a different kind of perception, a different kind of attitude in which our best qualities surface and briefly shine out from us.*

We experience this energy when we forgive somebody who's harmed or offended us, when we walk away from a gossip chorus, or pray for someone who's seriously ill. I remember reading a story about a man and a woman who were working in the same office. They didn't get along. They irritated one another constantly. One day the man said to her as they passed in the corridor: "That's a nice sweater. That blue looks really good on you." The antipathies dispersed like fog in the sun, and they became friends. Sometimes, walking down a crowded street, we may feel love for everyone we see, regardless of age, sex, race, social status etc. Here we are, crowds of us, crossing the road, strolling along the sidewalks, checking one another out, looking into store windows; each one of us with his or her unique memories, worries, hopes, joys, secrets…. and we all belong together.

When we are open to this feeling, a fine radiant energy travels through us like light passing through leaves or water. This energy, always alive in our being, is at the center of who we really are. The more we pay attention to it, the more we try to listen to it and follow the guidance it gives us, the more accessible it becomes, and the more we are able to watch things happen without being pushed up or down. We stay in the middle. We listen to the voices in ourselves saying: "I want this…. I can't live without that …" like kids in a toy store. And, like the kid's parent, we decide when to say yes, when to say no.

The Choice

If you can't say no, your yes doesn't mean much
—Diana Chornenkaya

I realized in Indonesia that everything I do matters. There are no days off from being me. Telling myself I'll straighten up next week, and meanwhile I'm going to get drunk or stoned again or have sex again with that girl/that guy just because I can and what the hell it won't make any difference in the long run it's not the end of the freaking world … this, to put it baldly, is a copout.

Much of the time we're in automatic mode, "asleep" as some call it, not really aware of what's going on. We can get through hours on automatic mode, sitting in classrooms, hanging out, stacking shelves, pumping iron or watching TV, and maybe all we've missed – though it's a lot! - is the experience of living fully in the present. But with sex the stakes are a lot higher. However casually we treat it sex is never casual, so – *and this is one of the hardest and most important tasks we can undertake* – ideally we struggle towards being able to make conscious choices about our sex lives. Because it's usually true that we can choose to have sex or not to have sex. (The major exception to this is if being raped, or drugged, or abused by someone bigger and more powerful. Also, if you're drunk or stoned, and don't know what's going on, although it's usually true that you chose to get drunk or stoned at some point.)

It's up to each one of us what we do with our bodies and sexual energies. Even if you're strongly aroused, you still have a choice. If you have sex without giving yourself time and space to choose, you've passed the decision over to your hormones, or to your need for acceptance, or to the fifth glass of wine. You're the ruler who has abdicated, making the throne available to the servants.

So then the question arises: *How do I make this choice?*

I'm trying to work out what it means to make a *conscious choice,* which means making a decision that's right for you. It may be a decision your partner doesn't like or agree with. It may even be a decision that *you* don't like. What we want and what's right for us don't always coincide. The thing is, once we start stepping back and reflecting on what's going on in our lives; once we start trying to make choices based on a sense of what we believe to be right for us rather than what we're used to or what we think will make the other person like or love us or because it's what everyone is doing… then we're waking up, we're becoming conscious, we're becoming a true human being.

Let's say you decide you're not going to have sex with your partner for…. two weeks. Maybe you reckon you've been going at it too much lately, and you want to cool things a bit. But then, you're making out and getting horny, and you think:

Oh I can't stand it…. I wanna do it!

So your body's pulling one way and your inner feeling is pulling the other, and you have a battle on your hands. You made a promise to yourself, and here you are panting like a race-horse, trying to forget that promise. This kind of battle - and its outcome - is very important. As you try to sort out and follow what's best for you, you define who you are. Or, as Jacob Needleman puts it "Everything *matters*. A man who sees or acts without primary reference to the inner power of will and intention is not a man." [1]

Let's look at a scenario:

So here's Dave Summerbee in his Mazda Miata, driving along the Santa Monica Freeway in LA. It's about 11.30 at night. In the passenger seat is Patricia Fernandez. Black hair light brown skin black halter top tight jeans.

They met at a beach party in Malibu two weeks ago… This is their second date. They've been to a club in Venice Beach. He's driving her home. She lives off Hollywood Blvd.

It's a beautiful night. The top's down. The summer air is cool on their faces. Another ten minutes or so and they'll be outside her house. Again. They were there last Saturday night, after a great dinner in a restaurant on Melrose. He was leaning across to kiss her and she put her hand on his cheek and said, "Thanks Dave" and opened the car door and walked up the path to her house.

That was last Saturday and this is 8 days later. Patricia has just told him she's a real strong Catholic and she's not into having sex with people. Yet. He wants to stop and put his arm along the back of the seat behind her head, and fill his fingers with her thick hair and turn her head so that she's facing him and he can look at her, 'cos he finds her totally gorgeous. And then lean forward and kiss her, and breathe in her fragrance and feel her mouth open and her hands twine around his neck.

"So... you don't sleep with guys?"

She shakes her head.

"Uhh uhh."

"You don't have sex."

"No."

"Not ever."

"One day I will."

"So... what do you date guys for? I mean, like, what do you WANT?"

Silence.

"Patricia?"

"Listen Dave if you don't wanna see me again because you can't have sex with me that's fine."

"Yeah. Right. Okay."

So there's Dave driving this gorgeous woman home.... and he's thinking:

How dare she turn me down man?

Doesn't she know the freaking SCORE?

I like her. I really like her. I like her a lot.

Over hundred bucks I've spent on this chick and ....

I'll work on her I'll keep working on her tell her can I come in for a moment grab a glass of water .....

How was I to know she was a Catholic..... damn!

Hey dude... think of this as a challenge.

If Dave were to turn to you, the reader, perched there on his shoulder as he signals for the turnoff, and say "What do I do?".... what would you say?

*Go for it man you've **earned** it*

Don't waste any more time on her

Play it cool. Kiss her on the cheek and drop her off and drive away like it's no big deal...

Depends what you want....

He likes her. He likes the way she laughs. And walks. And dresses. And talks. And smells. He likes who she is. If he comes on strong she'll probably close up on him.

If he accepts the relationship on her terms, he's letting her make the decisions about stuff he prefers to be in charge of. So Dave has a choice to make. He has a fight on his hands. Not with Patricia - although that could be seen as a contest - but with himself. This is a struggle about *who's the boss?* Not: is Dave the boss, or Patricia, but who's the boss inside Dave; which of the forces or voices inside him is he going to listen to? Which of them will influence him in a way that's best for him? And, of course, for her.

You may lose some of your innocence – or lack of awareness - about sexuality when you read this book. This is the kind of obliviousness that allows you to follow your impulses without thinking about the possible consequences. Like eating three double-decker hamburgers every week without worrying about chloresterol.

You can pretend to yourself that nothing's happening - even while you're involved in something that's happening. You can tell yourself that you're following your bliss when it's not bliss that you're following but pleasure. Or you can try to be clear about what's going on, so that you can *choose* what you're going to do, like the choice Dave has to make in his relationship with Patricia.

Most of us don't go around having casual sex all the time, or even most of the time. We fall in love.

And that, my friends, as you may know, is a tricky one.

Romantic love

I've kissed too many princes who turned into frogs
  – 17 year-old girl

I was sitting around with a bunch of young people in someone's kitchen talking about sex and so on and a young man called David said, "What about if you're in love?" At the time I had no good answer. Writing this book reminded me of his question, and of the story I'm about to tell:

I was working as a docker – longshoreman – at Folkestone harbor, on the coast of the English Channel. We used to sing as we unloaded crates and bales from a rusty old cargo boat and barrowed them into a big warehouse that stank of forklift diesel fumes, or braved the rain and the salty spray to heave luggage and bags of mail into railway wagons.

Up in Folkestone's expensive district there was a spacious art gallery called the Metropole Arts Center. It was run by a good friend of mine - John Eveleigh. One summer John organized an exhibition of art from both world wars. There were powerful paintings by famed British artists such as Graham Sutherland, Wyndham Lewis and John Piper. One day an unexpected spark jumped through my mind from the warehouse, where we were stashing bales of Italian cloth, and the Metropole Arts Center. I thought: "How about getting a bunch of us dockers together and singing war songs in the gallery, with all those great war paintings around?" When I described the idea to John he said, "Great idea! Why don't you do poems as well?"

About 10 dockers were up for it. We called ourselves "The Quaysiders." I found a pub pianist, and weekends we'd all gather round the big glossy grand in the gallery and sing old war songs:

> *Bless 'em all*
> *Bless 'em all*
> *The long and the sort and the tall*
> *You'll get no promotion*
> *This side of the ocean*
> *So cheer up my lads*
> *bless 'em all.*

I worked on finding poems with a wonderful theatrical couple - Donald Bain and Jesse Evans. I spent hours sitting in their big country house drinking single malt whisky and declaiming poems by Wilfred Owen and Siegfried Sassoon. I'd buzz home through the late-night Kentish lanes on my Vespa yelling Owen's Anthem for Doomed Youth at the sky, hearing startled cows thud away across the dark fields:

> *What passing bells for these who die as cattle?*
> *Only the monstrous anger of the guns*
> *Only the stuttering rifles' rapid rattle*
> *Can patter out their hasty orisons.*
> *No mockeries for them from prayers or bells*
> *Nor any voice of mourning save the choirs*

The shrill demented choirs of wailing shells
And bugles calling for them from sad shires.

In my head I was hearing a slow, jagged blues theme for the poem and needed a pianist to play it. Somebody introduced me to Barbara.

She was nineteen. Piano student at the Royal College of Music. Creamy skin, wide mouth, huge dark eyes, dark hair with a fringe. A fruity, breathy voice. I sang the bluesy tune I'd thought up for the Anthem. Slow walking bass, spiky melody. She got it after half an hour. The music and the feeling.

"The Pity of War" we called the show. The Quaysiders doing war songs, a rock group called The Nimbo J. Four doing Bob Dylan. Donald and Jessie reading poems. A clarinetist. A Japanese teenager reading a letter written to his mother apologizing for getting behind in his studies after the bomb dropped; his hair was falling out and he kept vomiting. The local newspaper featured a front-page photo of the Quaysiders in front of a huge painting by Wyndham Lewis of a WW1 first aid center. Someone pinned it up on the wall of the workman's canteen, and the Quaysider dockers walked with a certain swagger.

After rehearsals I'd take Barbara home on the scooter. We'd sit in the kitchen of her parents' house and talk about music, philosophy, mysticism. One night we drove to a cliff-top and sat looking at the lights of ships out on the Channel. I took her hand and stroked the soft warm skin of her palm and fingers. She trembled and whispered, "Stop..." but didn't take her hand away.

So it began.

It was intense.

One morning I drove to her house and walked through to the back garden. The French windows were open. Beethoven's seventh symphony on the stereo. It had rained in the night and everywhere drops of water were sparkling in the sun. Barbara was pruning roses. Liquid pearls gleamed on crimson and white petals. We were singing along with the music. I was watching lines of ants crossing and re-crossing the path. We entered then a dimension in which time seemed to be suspended. Light quivered and flashed. The green hills at the back of the town, the wide blue sky, the roses, the music, she and I ... everything was in a kind of timeless trance. It was an experience I shall never forget and never be able to satisfactorily describe.

Afterwards we both spoke of it; we were dazed and awed. We were completely and passionately in love.

A few weeks later we met in a little wood at the foot of the hills. It was raining fiercely, and we huddled together under a dripping tree. She seemed abstracted. Here in my arms, yet somewhere else. We made love on the wet leaves, big cold drops falling on to our skin. Afterwards she was crying. She pressed her head against my chest and whimpered, "It's not fair..." I didn't know what was going on. She wouldn't let me look into her eyes.

Not long after that, in the dockers' canteen, someone handed me a copy of the local newspaper. There was a notice announcing the engagement of Barbara Wilson to Brian Crabtree.

I was stricken. My world collapsed in on me. I didn't know what to do with the pain in my heart. I tried and tried to contact her, but by this time she was back in London and I had no idea how to find her. I got drunk, several times. Wrote sad poems:

So the morning closes round us
The waves sing on the beach

I pick at shells and fare-thee-wells
And you are out of reach.
Dragonflies and swallowtails
Pirouette and slice
Love is slowly dying
Like a trout beneath the ice

I drove back to the little wood below the hills one night and slept where we had lain together. My sleep was full of dreams; her face, her voice, her great dark eyes full of tears. I woke up aching and desolate, and drove home resolved to forget her.

Months passed. I was teaching in London. Took the train back to Folkestone for a weekend. Sunday evening, not knowing why, I decided to stay another day. Called my school principal. Caught the London train Monday evening. Walked through the empty compartment looking for a newspaper. Found Barbara, sitting alone.

"Hallo," she said in her breathy, slightly hesitant way. I sat opposite her.

She said our loving was so intense, so passionate, it was too much for her. When she was playing the piano she was playing for me. When I wasn't there she missed me. Missed us. Our love was taking her over. There was this Australian she'd met, another piano student at the Royal College of Music. He'd asked her to marry him. She thought they could play the piano together and be a normal couple and she could concentrate on her music. She'd had a dream in which she was trapped inside a piano and I was out there calling to her, and she was struggling to break through the strings.

I said she didn't love him. How could she marry him? I said I loved her, and I would never try to take her away from her music because it was such a big part of who she was, and anyway I loved music, so I would never expect or try to force her to choose. Our love was a force that would live and breathe and sing in her playing.

She cried piteously. I held her close and stroked her hair.

She said Brian was waiting at the station with his parents, who'd flown from Australia to meet her. We kissed and kissed. We kissed until we could hardly breathe. The train roared through the London suburbs. She said she would marry me if I'd be willing to leave England with her and go live somewhere else. She'd just disappear, not tell anyone, not even her parents. I said I had to think.

I researched English teaching jobs in France and Spain. Checked into visas and vaccination requirements. Checked what money I had in the bank. Then my inner told me to be careful. This could turn out to be bad. I told the whole story to an older friend, a Frenchman whose judgment I trusted. He shook his head, said it wouldn't work. Breaking a promise and running away was the wrong basis for a commitment. My heart cried No no no; my guts told me he was right.

Barbara and I met in a big park in the center of London. I said we can't do it like this. We have to be honest with everyone. Meet with Brian and his parents, and with her parents, and tell them a mistake's been made, that we love one another and want to be together. Otherwise the whole thing's wrong from the start.

She pleaded with me. "If you really loved me..." She was crying. She said she couldn't do it. I kissed her for the last time and walked away.

Years later I had a dream about us. I was standing at the window of a beautiful country house looking out across fields and woods. Suddenly a huge bird with two heads – one bearing my face, the other hers – swooped down and clutched me in its talons. It flew down and dived into the basement where it was dark and full of horrific whispering creatures.

When I awoke I knew that it would never have worked between us. I was freed, emptied of all longings for her.

What I understand from this is that romantic love, which is what we felt for one another, can be a truly blissful experience. But it's not real. It doesn't last. It's an enchantment. When Barbara pleaded with me to run away with her, leaving behind all the commitments and the promises and the people these were made to, it was like the story of the first lovers in Western literature, Tristan and Iseult, who loved one another despite the fact that Iseult was married to the king, and who left behind all that was "right" and "dutiful" and fled to the forest to be with one another. They spent three years living on nuts and berries, shivering in the rain and cold.

The Barbara I loved was a kind of dream princess; in fact, I called her "Princess Appassionata", (the Appassionata being the title of the Beethoven piano sonata she was learning when we met). She got engaged because she was seeking a relationship that was more "normal", less intense, less consuming. When she did this I was stricken. My Princess had deceived me. She had lain in my arms and loved me in the cold English rain even as she was planning to marry another.

The truth is, I never knew who she really was. She was beautiful, and a brilliant pianist, and had an elusive, shy-deer-in-the-woods quality that drew me to her, but it was just a dream I had, and I'm grateful to my wise French friend for waking me up and saving me from running off into the forest with her, leaving behind outraged parents and a pile of broken promises, depending on love and little else to see us through. The message delivered by the bird with two heads was that, when the enchantment ended – as it always does – and we saw one another as we really were, we would have been left facing a disaster.

The paradox is this: We may not know what true happiness is until we find love, and we may not know true pain until we lose it. If someone else were to ask me "What if you're in love?" I might tell the story of Barbara and me, and then say: *Don't give all of yourself to romantic love. Try not to let romantic love become the center of your life. If you do, you may be devastated when the spell breaks- as it always does – and you leave the enchanted kingdom. You will remember all the promises and the passion, and you will feel devastated; you will feel as though life has deceived you.*

WHAT'S RIGHT FOR ME

Nature, Mr. Alnut, is what we are put on earth to rise above.
- Katherine Hepburn, in the movie The African Queen.

Years ago I was teaching College English south of LA. I used to enjoy going beyond the instructor role and just talking with students as human beings. One of my English 101 students – a gorgeous black girl – told me one day that she was a virgin. The next day, quite coincidentally, another student in another class – told me *she* was a virgin. "You girls should get together," I joked. "Start a support group for virgins."

To my surprise they did. They called it the V Club. Soon they had about 10 members, mostly – but not all – female. Then they asked me and Amelia to be associate members of an offshoot group called 'Quandaries Anonymous.'

Quandaries Anonymous. I don't remember who came up with it, but it was a wonderful idea. Make a great movie. The way it worked was this: if you were out on a date and you were getting really horny you could – *if you chose to* – call Q.A. for help:

"Listen you guys I'm on a date with this total, like, hunk... I'm in the foyer of the multiplex waiting for him to drive to the front in his dark green Porsche and pick me up... and he is SO like totally SMOOTH and I just need you to like tell me again what I said about the virginity thing... 'cos things are like warming up over here and I need some help..."

Do we have the equivalent of Q.A. in our heads? Is there a part of ourselves that will pick up the phone when we call, and remind us again of the promise we made to ourselves as the great sweet tide of desire urges at us? Can we control our sexual feelings so that they don't dominate us, so that they don't force us into to satisfying them? Sex is part of a complex bigger picture, and I think it would be useful to have a quick look at some of this bigger picture. So we're going off the immediate subject of sex for a while. Please stay with me.

We start by considering choice, voice and conscience.

I used to think God made a big mistake in giving us choice. *"We should have some kind of implant in our heads that administers a jolt when we choose wrongly,"* I told him. *"You could do it. Kind of celestial microchip. Think of all the trouble that would save. And make the jolt more painful if we ignore the first one and go ahead anyway."* Most of us know somehow what's right for us, not only because of what we've been told by parents, teachers, ministers etc, but also because, beneath all the other monologs and dialogs going on within us all the time, we have a voice deep inside us. Can I say what I mean by this "voice"? No, not precisely; you could think of it as what we hear when someone really speaks from their "place of truth', or from their inner. I hear it occasionally in a poem by a child or a teenager. Here's a story that points towards what I mean:

A few years ago Andy, an old friend, called me up from his home about 300 miles away and said he needed to talk. He sounded really upset. He turned up the next day and told me his story.

He was sitting in a coffee bar in San Francisco when he noticed an attractive woman in her early twenties at another table. She was reading a book by a writer he liked, so he used this as a starting point for conversation, and soon he was sitting at her table getting to know her. They got on well and he was strongly attracted to her. After a while they decided to leave. As he held the door to the coffee bar open and she walked out past him, he heard a voice inside him say loudly and clearly:

"You're going to regret this. Say goodbye now!"

Meanwhile he was checking out her body and feeling horny, so he said, "Get lost!" to the voice and followed her out.

Soon after this meeting they started sleeping together. He said it was so intensely passionate he couldn't stay away from her.

One evening – as usual – he went to her apartment and rang the bell. There was no response. He rang again and waited. Nothing. He went back to the street, found a phone booth and dialed her number. No reply.

He went home, came back to her street, tried her apartment again, rang her number. No answer. He felt sick in his heart.

The next day there was a letter from her. It said: " Andy – I've gone to live in San Diego. Please don't come looking for me. I don't want to see you again. Goodbye. Carol"

Andy and I drove to the sea and lit a fire on the beach and he talked and talked and cried and talked and asked questions neither of us had any answers to. He read the letter over and over again, as though there were some hidden meaning that he might have missed. He was in a terrible state. Because I'd been there myself I felt a lot of compassion for him. "I should have listened to my voice," he said, over and over again.

In the end he read the letter one last time and, with a huge sigh, threw it in the fire. Then he drove home and carried on with his life.

Part of my sitting-by-the-white-wall experience was a gradual hushing of the superficial voices yammering away inside me. I didn't really know anything about life, I realized, except that I loved kids and loved working with them. Maybe at heart I was still a kid. A kid with an adult body and adult desires. Who am I? Don't know. How can I make choices that are right for me? Don't know. What does my life mean? Don't know. Every thought I had struck me as absolute codswallop. Where did that come from? What's the matter with you? Who are all these voices in me, blabbering away? Shut up shut up SHUT UP! Later I wrote this:

The squatters

Somewhere in the middle of this motley crowd
there's you.... the one for whom this place
was originally intended. Most of these characters moved in
when you first took over. Without so much as a
by your leave I might add. Built their own extensions
blocked out windows, added new ones, made drastic alterations
in the landscaping, changed the whole FEEL of the place.
It didn't stop at that let me tell you.
If any of them wanted something
they'd make damn sure they got it. You'd be amazed.
Moods. Dreams. That death wish you've been getting lately....

it's not you. So don't for goodness sake
give in to it. Clothes. Music. Drugs. You put a stop to
that thank God.
Alcohol. Women. Oh my goodness me yes.
No wonder so many of them were against
your getting married. I still don't understand
quite how you managed that.
Particularly after they made such a mess of your first one.
  The sad thing is
you still don't know they're there. They're clever, yes,
one has to
hand it to them. Subtle. You won't like this, but the
fact is
they manipulate you. ALL THE TIME. You still think
you have the whole place to yourself. It would be funny
if it weren't all such a shame. I've been here for years
trying to get through to you. Awful job, to be quite honest.
Sometimes I wish I'd never....
but that's another story.
  Lately you've been sitting in the garden with your
  eyes closed.
For hours at a time. I think you're listening.
Everybody scuttles off and hides of course
when they see you doing this. Everyone but me that is.
I run around taping messages on doors and windows:
"there's one in here..." "there's one in here...."
And now... today.... at last ....I've managed to get
through to you
to write all this. Yes my friend, it's true.
So read this carefully
when we've finished. And please don't be afraid.
We'll get these layabouts out of here. Promise. I won't
leave
until it's done. Actually, I can't.
But that's another story.

Our inner voice can cut through all the static and tell us truths we may not want to hear, like the message Andy ignored as he held the café door open inhaling Carol's aura. Let's go back to Dave Summerbee. He's driving home after dropping Patricia off.

He feels like he's in a kind of atmosphere, or bubble or something that's made up of all the impressions and feelings and sounds and smiles and scents and movements of Patricia. It surrounds him, fine as waves of music. Simultaneously he's suffering from a severe case of blue ball. He's thinking that Patricia is a special lady, and the phrase "special lady" somehow works loose and unpeels, like a label from a jar of sweet rich honey. He says her name: "Patricia" out loud. He says, out loud, "I love her." He's not sure why he said this, or what it means. He loves the quality of her. It's so … it's fine. It's that fineness in her that he's touched by, even though it's what prompts her to say "No" when he comes on at her, and it's that fineness that leads him to accept her "No" even though he wants her so fiercely her it feels like his blood is about to burst. He tells himself he wants to be with her even though she won't have sex with him. In fact, in a way, he wants to be with her because she won't have sex with him, partly – and I think only partly – because he wants her so badly the thought of not having her is worse than anything he can think of, and if he stops seeing her because he can't have her now he'll never have her. I think that's what's going on in him. He has the feeling that when they finally make love it will blow the top of his head off. At least. He drives off the freeway and sits there for a while. "What the f…'s going on ?" Never has his heart been touched so deeply.

Inside Dave there's an awakening going on. He's going through his version of my sitting by the white wall experience; old habits, patterns, expectations are losing their grip on him, and as the space quietens down the voice of Dave is – faintly at first – to be heard. Love can do that to you.

Voice and Conscience

I'm still working on this, but I think of voice as the inner side of conscience, and conscience as the sense of what's right for me and for others which, with the exception of psychopaths, is common to us all. Conscience is a mix of our own masculine and feminine energies, both of which, ideally, are at work in us in more or less equal partnership. Masculine, or fatherly conscience insists that there must be consequences to wrongdoings and that love must be deserved. Feminine, or motherly conscience is the voice of unconditional love, a love that no hurt or crime can diminish. If the fatherly conscience is too dominant, we will judge ourselves – *and others* – harshly and unforgivingly, like the preacher dispatching sinners to eternal fires. If the motherly conscience is too dominant we will be so non-judgmental that we – *and others* – will live in a chaotic, "anything goes" dimension.

When the two are balanced then, whether we're male or female, we are able to develop and articulate clear standards, or values, to live by, but can forgive ourselves when we don't attain them. If we can balance these two qualities – motherly and fatherly – in our relationship with ourselves, then we can carry this over into our relationship with others. Our capacity for tenderness and empathy is balanced by our capacity for reason and order. This may be one of the definitions of mature love.

Yes I love you
I love you as you are
But not all that you do
Is right
I accept who you are
But I do not have to accept
Everything you do

Talking to our conscience

Sitting by the white wall I wondered how I might have avoided some of the mistakes I'd made. We like to think of mistakes as opportunities for learning, and of course they are. But I realized it's not as simple as that. I met a crazy American in Cilandak, someone who, oddly enough, had known some of my old London friends and who'd done a lot of the same stuff I had. He was a rangy, ambling man who walked, as I told him one day, like a two-legged horse. He used to come by and rave about Lord of the Rings-type visions he'd had of dragons flying over the River Thames with light-filled eggs in their jaws. He took me along a path one afternoon and said," Stop! Now, look around. Really carefully." I saw a fence. Rice paddies on the other side of it, and Indonesian houses beyond them made of rattan and bamboo. Palm trees in front of me, to the left of the path. Ah! What was that? A little twinkle of light. There, on the knobbly trunk. "You saw it man!" He'd stuck a thumb tack in the trunk, and at a certain angle, at a certain time of the day, if you were looking in the right direction, it flashed at you as you walked along the path.

"That's deep," I told him.

"Best thing I ever did," he said.

One day, very unusually, he sat with me in silence for a long time, then started, quite quietly, to cry. He said he'd screwed up his life, and didn't think he'd ever find his way back to God. He didn't want to talk about what he'd done, about how he'd screwed up – he said that brought it all back. He said screwing up was human, and God forgave us. But when we know we're screwing up and we go on doing it anyway, then we lose touch with God.

I said I didn't think God was going anywhere. He shook his head violently, almost angrily, and said we can make it a lot harder for ourselves if we're trying to find our way back to God. When you've wasted time screwing around, he said, *especially when you know you're screwing around*, nothing you can do will bring that time back.

I was wishing I had the spiritual stature to lay my hand on his shoulder and say, truthfully and for real: "You are forgiven". He was intense and loony, but I was touched by what he said about finding his way to God, and I knew that, however hard it got, both of us were lucky to have ended up in this humid purgatorial enclave, far from old habits, safe from the craziness of London.

Maybe in a way he was right. Clearly there's a difference between doing something that's harmful to yourself and maybe others without knowing that it's harmful, and doing the same thing *knowing* that it's harming yourself and others.

I had no idea, back in my primrose path days, that there were spiritual consequences to having sex. Once I became aware of these consequences everything changed. I was – and am – still free to do what I want, but now I know the score. Growing up means – among other things – becoming aware of the consequences of what we do. It's a loss of innocence. Reading this book may take away some of your innocence about sex.

Sorry about that.
Not.

There's a story I heard about Adam – how he'd originally been in spirit form, zooming around in time and space borne by the momentum of his wishes, complete freedom being the name of the game. Then God told Adam he wanted to give him a body and a new home, called earth. Naturally, Adam balked at this idea, but God reassured him and told him his new home had everything he needed and that he'd be very happy there, provided he remembered who had created him and the earth. If he forgot he'd be in trouble. So Adam said okay, I'll give it a whirl, or words to that effect. Came here and loved the place so much he kept forgetting.

What did it mean: "…find my way back to God?" I had no idea who or what God was. God's more real to me now, but at the time I needed something a bit closer to home. "Find my way back to me" seemed more accessible. Perhaps, in the end, it would amount to the same thing.

WHO AM I?

The search for this sense of self… is a spiritual journey because it inevitably results in the discovery that our greatest wisdom lies within. We may learn from teachers and read great books, but ultimately each of us must learn to trust our inner wisdom.

– Harville Hendrix

Even in my partially deconstructed state I'd noticed that the people I met in Cilandak – the Americans, the Dutch, the Indonesians, the Germans, the Japanese, the English and the French – were more strongly themselves than people I'd known before. When I talked to anyone there I had the feeling that he or she wasn't trying to impress me, or judge me, or hide behind some role or style they'd spent years formulating. They were simply themselves, being who they were. It made social interactions a bit tricky for me; I couldn't do the old routines the thickly bearded me in the passport photo was familiar with, but I still hadn't managed to sort out who I really was, so socially I was in limbo and, for a while, rather inept.

Now I want to jump a lot of years from then to now, from the verandah by the hot white wall to this table with its computer, its lamp and its view of hills and pale houses and evening-darkened North Californian sky. Here's what I think about who we are. This may change; in fact, I hope it will. I often remind myself to consider all my beliefs in as incomplete and all my conclusions as statements of the past.

I remember, about 17 years ago, holding in my arms a tiny lightweight bundle that kicked little legs and opened tiny eyes and made a weak, high-pitched crying sound. I was holding my daughter, Davina, just born, minutes into the world. I was so moved I was laughing and crying at the same time. I felt as though I was holding a miracle.

Birth is a miracle. I mean by birth the whole cycle of human conception, the growth of the embryo in the mother's womb, and the process of delivery, of emergence into this world. It's a miracle that you and I and every human being in the world originate from.

I believe that the process of growing from sperm and egg to embryo to baby is master-minded by the human force working with the raw materials provided by the mother. This force enters the womb through the union of sperm and egg and begins building a home for itself, a physical body with everything it will need for its life on earth.

This soul, with its urge to live here in the world, is who we are. It's our original nature. So it could be said that we are most purely ourselves when we are babies. This may seem a little strange. Bear with me.

What happens to the baby? It grows and grows and learns and learns. It works at moving its limbs and looking and listening and making sounds; it takes in fuel, sleeps, wakes to work some more. It learns to recognize its mother, then other family members. It learns to crawl and walk, to eat pulped banana, to pick things up. It learns what tastes bad, what sunlight feels like, and warm water, and cat fur. It explores its world continuously, and its world gets bigger and bigger.

Babies and toddlers learn all this without being taught. We all learnt how to do these things, in our own ways, in our own times, not because we consciously wanted to, but because the human energy moved us to. We worked at learning because this fulfilled our purpose.

As we get older our world becomes more complicated. The people around us begin teaching us things. Our mother teaches us, our father teaches us, other family members teach us. They all influence us. Then we go to school and teachers teach us. Our peers teach us, or influence us. We are taught, or shaped, by our culture – by TV programs, internet, video games, films, books, comics, songs, sports, and so on.

As all these influences enter our lives we lose more and more of our capacity to follow this original, human energy that shapes us in the womb and guides us when we leave it. We change from being 'natural' children to being 'normal' children, and our original true self is covered over by more and more layers.

This process is called socialization.

As in 'The Squatters', it's as though our house – our inner space – is invaded by wave after wave of other people, each with their version of how the house should be run, while we, the original tenants, find ourselves being so crowded out that we end up crouching in the basement or the attic. So by the time we reach our late teens most of us have lost touch with who we really are. In their efforts – well-meant, in most cases – to teach us to fit in, our caretakers – parents, teachers, counselors etc. – blur our uniqueness and dilute our spontaneity.

Jacob Needleman's description of "our bric-a-brac minds" echoes this idea: "Our bric-a-brac mind is constantly serving us up its furnishings, pictures and appliances in all their disconnected dusty glory. Yet very few, if any, of these ideas, views and opinions that color and shape our experience and our very lives have ever been examined and weighed as to their truth and worth. Very rarely, if ever, are we even aware of them. We are, perhaps, never aware that this or that passion or decision or anxiety or hope or resolute action is not "mine" at all, but actually belongs to some disconnected idea, view or opinion that has taken up lodging in my mind and is actually doing my "thinking" for me. It is not *I* who take this passionately held moral stance, let us say, and am ready to sacrifice my all for it, it is an appliance in my mind that *feels* like *me*, only because my real self, has never stepped forward to look at it, examine it, and decide whether to keep it and use it."[1]

The good news is: however repressive our childhood and early youth and however crazy our teens and early adulthood, *nothing can stop us finding our way back to wholeness if this is what we choose to do.* Finding this 'way back' to our true self is one of our central life tasks. Part of this task lies in recognizing what holds us back on this quest.

Because nearly all of us are subjected to this socialization process we rarely meet anyone who wasn't, so we have no standard of comparison. The people I met in Cilandak were, as I said, more strongly themselves than most. When you do meet someone who's 'natural' rather than 'normal', the difference is obvious. The drum they follow is their own, beating their own rhythm.

I've spent most of my life teaching in schools, and have concluded that teachers and administrators – sincere, hard-working people by and large – don't know that they're holding young people back from understanding who they are or what their talents are.

We probably need other people to teach us skills. We learn how to walk by ourselves, but it's harder to learn calculus or auto repair or karate or a foreign language without someone there to pass on their skills. Because teachers have to "teach to the test", students are often forced to learn stuff they're not ready to learn and have little or no interest in. So most young people go through years of schooling in a half-switched off state, and their soul, or inner self – the "book in our chest", as it's been described – is so covered up it's almost beyond reach. This makes it very hard for us to develop an inner sense of what's right for us, and what's wrong. For this reason there are benefits for young people in belonging to a religion. It will provide them with a clear moral or ethical code, and a support system, guidelines that protect them until they are strong and clear enough to develop their own.

We are all born with everything we need within us to grow and learn in ways that are right for us and live fulfilling, productive lives. The package we're given includes our talents, which lead us towards the work that's right for us. If our schools, colleges and universities don't nourish our awareness of our talents, the chances are we'll step out into the world in our teens or twenties with no clear sense of purpose.

The good news is: Who we really are is still alive inside us. The soul cannot be destroyed, and it never stops calling us back to our wholeness. Old stories often tell of an 'awakening', in which some force awakens the main character from sleep and brings him/her to full awareness and life. Movies like "The Truman Show" and "The Matrix" tell of characters who discover that the life they've been leading is a kind of sleep, or dream,

Much of what's going on in the teens and twenties has to do with trying out identities as we seek an answer to this 'Who am I?' question. This search for selfhood involves distancing yourself from your parents to prove to yourself that you're no longer their child. We may define ourselves by rebelling against them and by attacking or criticizing one or more of the following:

teachers, preachers, principals, politicians, celebrities, bosses, cops, anyone over 65, 30, or 21, people who shop at Wal Mart, people who don't smoke dope, white people, Hispanics, people with a lot of money, men with hairy bodies, women with hairy armpits, Republicans, pole dancers, Democrats, people in uniforms, wealthy people who wear torn jeans, rednecks, gays, feminists, activists, anarchists, Christians, carnivores, men who swagger, lumberjacks, people who shoot defenseless animals, society as a whole.

Some young people, pushed by anger and/or by a raw need for connection and love, become highly promiscuous, and I always feel sad when I see this happening. I understand the needs, but also I know that promiscuity messes us up inwardly. Seeking love or relatedness by sleeping around results only in superficial connections that leave us feeling more cut off. Seeking to define ourselves by sleeping around opens our inner door to strangers and blurs our sense of who we are and therefore makes it harder for us to define ourselves.

I went through hell in my teens. Towards the end, as things got better, I vowed that when I became an adult I would do whatever I could to make things a little less difficult for other teenagers and young people. I've tried to do that in lots of ways, this book being one of them.

Hang in there. Stay in the middle. It gets better. It gets better.

The Vacuum

"At the innermost core of all loneliness is a deep and powerful yearning for union with one's lost self"
— Brendan Francis

W e were in a kind of leisure center on the seaward side of Jakarta. There was a winding tiled canal about 70 yards long that looped around past outdoor cafes and under bridges. The water was comfortably cool and flowing. You could lie on your back and gently paddle your hands and feet and drift beneath the tropical sky, expending little effort, floating beneath the same bridges and smiling at the people you passed not long ago. I remember an English friend saying, as she drifted past me, "It's quite like living in Indonesia really, isn't it?"

In many ways it was an accurate simile. In Indonesia – or at least in Java, the part of Indonesia I came to know quite well – the basic social unit is the group. Prod one Javanese and twenty quiver. So Indonesians are rarely alone, and rarely lonely. I used to go off for long walks in the mountains, and the locals would approach me with a smile me and say: "Jalan-jalan sendirian tuan ...?" – *off for a walk by yourself?* For them it was a very strange thing to do. In the West for the past four or five hundred years the basic social unit has been the individual. I'm not suggesting that one's better than the other, but it is true to say that there are millions of lonely people in the West. As individuals we gain in qualities like initiative, innovation, independence, risk-taking etc. But we lose in terms of community and the qualities and elements that come with community, like a sense of belonging, of togetherness, of roots and rituals. As far as I could see the Javanese were happy to be together in this warm laughing gently-teasing continuum. It gave them the feeling that they had enough.

Many of us Westerners live with a sense of emptiness, of something missing. To some extent this is a natural result of growing up. We define ourselves by separating ourselves from our parents. Simultaneously there's an inner separation happening. We're evolving beyond the simple wholeness of childhood. Remember how spontaneous and immediate life was when you were a kid? As Salamah says: *The child's once fully conscious psyche is slowly dividing into conscious and unconscious areas of his or her mind ... This is the stage of 'the divided self', the existential vacuum, the 'emptiness within'. It is not a comfortable stage and it may last a long time.*

In addition to this inner process there are three outer factors contributing to this sense of emptiness:

1. The endlessly repeated message that happiness is to be found in buying lots of things,
2. The socialization process described earlier, which tends to bury our true self, and
3. The absence of the coming of those age rituals practiced in traditional societies that express the young person's separation from family and

emergence into the larger community with a new social and spiritual identity.

(For more on ritual see Colin Turnbull's book "The Human Cycle". For more on the emergence of the "Self" see Barbara Ehrenreich's brilliant book "Dancing in the Streets".)

In the West, marriage used to be the ritual that brought us into responsible adulthood, but it's largely lost this powerful, central significance. Young people, as a result, are given very little help in trying to find out who they are, mainly because this journey towards self-discovery simply isn't acknowledged in any meaningful communal *ritual*. The need is still there, strong as ever, but society – through its education system – trains young people to be citizens, workers and consumers – all outer roles – and pays scant heed to their inner need for some kind of meaningful rite of passage.

Here's a poem showing the thoughts of a teenager being lectured by an adult authority figure:

My own good
You're older than me. More powerful.
You've organized the world in such a way
that if I do not do what you expect of me
you tell me that I've failed, and make me feel it.

I make myself believe you. It's easier.
If I question your expectations and requirements
and try to tell you why I question them
you make a 'rebel' of me. That's not the issue.

You control the world. The world
is where I live. And so I tell myself
it's easier to give in to you

play the game according to your rules.

What choices do I have? Sometimes I try to follow
what I want to follow
do what I feel moved to do, according to
my sense of who I am, of what's right for me.

If I don't, I won't know who I am.
And if I don't know who I am
how can I live my life, how can I know
that what I do is me, that this is why I'm here?

There may be moments when you smile wryly
and look back through the years
and say, "I used to feel like that
a long long time ago."

And you might wonder when things changed
what was gained and what was lost.
And when you do, perhaps at last
we will be able to talk to one another.

The good thing about the vacuum (or whatever we want to call it) is that it may set us off on a journey, or a quest. This quest, which begins in adolescence and continues through the twenties and even further, could be defined as *the search for who I really am.*

Recently I read a poignant extract from "The Price of Privilege" by Madeline Levine, a clinical psychologist in which she describes having a conversation with a 15 year-old girl who had used a razor to carve the word EMPTY on her forearm. It can be really difficult, living through your teens or twenties with this vacuum inside you. You may be under insistent pressure from your parents and teachers to work hard at school, get high grades, get into a good college… etc. You may be busy creating a persona (like the caddis grub) so that you can fit in, have friends, be accepted, make a place for yourself in school or college or wherever. You may find definition through a relationship: *"This person really wants to be with me… this person makes me feel like I belong, like I matter, like I'm someone who's worthy of love."*

And, yes, such feelings are strong and seal over that sense of emptiness and make you feel wonderful. But the truth that's really hard to believe while you're in the middle of this joy is that it's a mistake to depend completely on another person to define and substantiate us. Here's Julia, an Australian girl, trying to sort out her feelings about a relationship that had just ended:

I've been feeling lately that Phillip is the cause of my sadness – I loved him, I did feel that he loved me. We were very much part of each other and wanted to be, so I thought. Then he dumped me.

Maybe he's not the real cause of my sadness. He was filling my inner vacuum, hence filling my life. In fact, he was filling it with so much stuff that it kept me from developing any more of my own stuff. It also made it more difficult at times for me to recognize my own stuff. That was fine with me because I could concentrate on him and I didn't, couldn't develop any more of my own … so really I am the cause of my sadness.

WHY ON EARTH DO I DO THIS TO MYSELF?

So we were both concentrating on him and I lost hold of myself and when he left me I felt like an idiot because the whole time I was concerning myself with him a little voice was yelling "What about me?"

What I did was tell that voice "You'll be fine. He needs me now; he's confused, helpless. It's my job to look after him and when I've helped him to understand, loved him and stood by him he'll love me back"

Then he dumped me.

So now I'm left with the inner voice saying, "But.... he didn't love me back. Why? Aren't I worth loving?"

That's the big question after someone dumps you: "Aren't I worth loving?"

The sad thing for a lot of people is that after a few failed relationships they start to believe they're not worth loving, and subconsciously go about attracting others with the same underlying belief/fear and consequently set themselves up for another difficult tragic fall.

If you're lucky your parents didn't pressure you too much when you were a kid. If they gave you limits *and* freedom and unconditional love then you were less pulled away from who you are and you won't have to fight so hard to retrieve your sense of self. If, however, they repressed, ignored or abused you, then your real nature went 'underground', and you'll have a lot more work to do. This will probably include a lot of acting out. The more repressed you were as a child, the more you have to struggle as a teenager and young adult to throw off the layers of 'stuff' around you. (For more on this see Alice Miller's book: "For Your Own Good." Also the IPC website "The Process Works.") To be fair, if your parents are like this, the chances are they're repeating what happened to them when they were children.

If you were harshly repressed, or physically or sexually abused, then the pain that you experience can be so intense that you may look for an escape through sex, drugs, alcohol, petty crime, or violence. Trouble is, these escapes may destroy you. (And, quite possibly, others.)

The bottom line then is this:

*To find out who you are you may have to 'act out', or rebel. But you may rebel in a way that harms you and make it harder for you to find out who you really are. Whatever's going on, however bad it gets, **you must look after yourself.***

Alternatively you may put all your energies into playing the game that your parents and society seem to expect of you, and put a lot of effort into school work, achieving self-esteem through high grades and academic success. There's nothing wrong with this, of course, except that it may have little to do with who you really are. I know a gifted young English woman, Louise, who was an 'A' student through high school and for nearly three years at art college. Then, in her early twenties, she suddenly dropped out. She said, "*I got fed-up with being a frigging 'A' student. That wasn't who I was.*"

Louise needed to find out for herself who she was in terms of work, community, relationship and children, and she found the courage to do this. Many of the teenagers who drop out of high school are doing the same thing at an earlier age.

For some the journey continues beyond this. If work – and marriage or long-term relationship – lose some of their glow, we may wonder: What else is there? I remember Barbara telling me how her father, who'd worked hard for years to become manager of an upper-class men's clothing store, got up one morning and sat at the top of the stairs overcome by a feeling that it had all been a complete waste of time. It was all completely futile. His doctor prescribed pills and a two-week holiday. It's been said that if we ignore messages like this we remain on the limited fate level. If we ponder them and try to act on what they're telling us, we transcend our fate and fulfill our destiny, which is to become a true human being.

One of my college students, a writer of painfully perceptive stories, told me that she often feels like an outline of a person, like a sketch for an unfinished picture. Her lungs function, and her digestive system, and her blood and brain and so on, but they're all working away to maintain a kind of shell, a gap with skin around it, and clothes. She only feels real when a man wants to have sex with her or is having sex with her. She's afraid of being alone because then she feels as though she doesn't really exist, but when she's with a man she gets so needy and clingy she ends up driving him away and she's back to being alone again. She said she thought some of this emptiness came from her childhood, which was, to use her word, "shitty". But she also thought that maybe there was something else, a deeper need. Sex helped her feel better for a while, but it didn't fulfill this need, so she was going to go celibate and try to figure out what was really going on. "I'm gonna jump in the hole," she told me," and see where I end up."

Sex can make us feel alive, or at least less dead. This is why it can be such a compelling force. But it is an experience that makes us – in ways that we have talked about – open to the energies in the other person. Loving ourselves means protecting ourselves from harm, so before we have sex with someone we might ask ourselves:

Is this the right thing to do?

Do I really want to do this?

Will making love with this person help me feel good about myself?

Am I certain that this person truly loves and respects me?

Does being with this person bring me closer to myself, closer to other people, and (maybe) closer to God?

And...(maybe the hardest one of all) what do I sense about this person's Basic Level Of Being?

Questions like these are to do with what our values are. My value system back in the primrose path days, was, as I said: *If it feels nice, do it.* Seemed okay at the time. Later I saw that for me it was totally inadequate.

Values

Talk of values, of stopping on the brink of sex to ask oneself a series of rather solemn questions may seem like a real downer. Feel free to skip this section if you think you've got things worked out he said with a quizzical smile. For the rest of you... here goes.

By values I mean the ethics that each of us lives by. They're a handrail for us to clutch when hormones are dancing us around the dizzy maypole. They have their uses. There's a core of values that's recognized pretty well globally. Here's a quick list:

There's a value that speaks of love, of reverence for life – human and non-human. It says that we should not harm or hurt one another.

There's a value that speaks of honesty, or truthfulness. It says that we should not lie to one another, or to ourselves.

There's a value that speaks of generosity, of empathy towards the needs of others. It says that we should leave enough for others, whether they are our contemporaries or our descendants.

There's a value that speaks of freedom. It says that we should be free to make choices in our lives, and that we shouldn't limit the freedom of others unless they are disturbing or inconveniencing us.

And there's a value that speaks of individual purpose. It says that we are born with talents, and with a capacity for love, for making the world a better place. It says that our task is to discover these capacities and fulfill them.

These values, and others, are familiar to most of us. If we could really live by them our world would be a radically better place. Most of us achieve some of them some of the time; probably all of us could do a better job of this.

Because we rarely see positive values being followed in the world, it's easy to dismiss them as irrelevant. When there's a war going on somewhere every day; when the physical condition of our planet is deteriorating every day; when thousands of people die of hunger and disease every day… it's hard to believe that these values make any difference.

Being human means continuing to try.

Wars go on breaking out, but hundreds of thousands of people go on working for peace.

The planet goes on deteriorating, but hundreds of thousands of people continue to commit themselves to halting and reversing this process of deterioration.

People continue to die of hunger and disease… and others among us go on committing their lives to helping and healing them.

Real values are those that we work out for ourselves, or those we somehow come across and think *'Yes, that's true!'* When values are *out there*, like slogans delivered by leaders, teachers, preachers, etc. – they're not much good to us, even if they're true.

Values are only of value when they're alive inside us.

Living according to values may seem hard and joyless. The fact is, evolving values and doing our best to stay true to them helps us to feel good about ourselves.

Here's a memorable insight from psychologist David J. Lieberman:

"… when you make a choice to do what is right, you feel good about yourself. This is because to feel good you must do good. Only when you are able to choose responsibly are you in charge of your life and do you gain self-respect. Then your actions are free and you feel good about yourself. …. So we see that doing what is right nourishes our psyche. You gain self-respect and in turn self-esteem. That is how self-respect and self-control are intertwined." [1].

How do values relate to sex?

They have to do with how you feel about your body and your own being, what kind of relationship you're looking for, what would make it right for you to have sex with someone.

They have to do with your understanding of what sex *means.*

– is it mainly a physical act or is it the expression of a deep feeling of love?

– is it something you do so that your partner will love you?

– is it something you do because pretty well everyone you know is doing it and you want to appear cool?

We all need to be loved. This is natural, and potentially positive. But if our values are vague and our needs urgent, we may make unwise compromises to gain this love. *"If you love me I will feel better about myself. What can I do to make you love me?"* Values help us when we're being tugged at like this. If we know what's right for us then, as I said earlier, we have a handrail to hold on to, and this is much better than vaguely hoping that things will turn out okay, or not even allowing ourselves to think about what we're doing.

Yes, all this is much more easily said than done. You can have strong clear values, and then you meet someone and find yourself so powerfully attracted you toss your values out the window and just go ahead. Maybe the guy's married and has kids but you really have the hots on for him. Or it's a girl who's torn up because her boyfriend has just ditched her, and you're comforting her, and then you come on at her when all she really wanted was to be held...

Working out our values and making choices that are in tune with them helps us feel that we are in charge of what's going on. We develop inner strength. We start to define – to ourselves and to others – who we are, what we stand for. Not giving ourselves a hard time when we blow it is important. If we can learn to forgive ourselves we'll travel a lot more lightly. Amelia, my bee-keeper wife, showed me this poem:

> *Last night as I was sleeping*
> *I dreamt, oh marvelous error*
> *That I had a beehive*
> *Here inside my heart*
> *And the golden bees*
> *Were making white combs*
> *And sweet honey*
> *From my old failures.*
>
> - Antonio Machado, trans. Robert Bly

The following quote is about teenagers but is, I believe, true for all of us:
On the way to wise decision- making teenagers go through different levels of understanding and, ultimately, maturity:

Level 1. Teenagers do not struggle with making a tough choice

Level 2. Teenagers play back their memories of decisions made and acknowledge what they did wrong

Level 3: Teenagers recognize a bad decision when they are in the act of deciding but feel powerless to make a different decision

Level 4: Teenagers identify a decision as a bad one before they act on it and choose an alternative. [5]

What helps us assess a decision – or an impulse! – as to whether it's good or bad is, surely, our sense of values. Often we just go along with what's happening because it's what other people are doing and if they're all doing it it's probably okay. Each one of them is no doubt thinking some version of the same thing. It can be hard to stop and say No when everyone's going on and saying Yes. That was why I went to Cilandak. Back in London I knew I had to stop doing stuff because it was harming me, but all my friends were doing the same stuff as I was, so if I wanted to stop doing the stuff I was doing I had to get away from them, hard though it was.

Older people like me run on a lot about sex, but in the end it's what *you* think and feel, what *you* work out and decide for yourself, that counts. I do urge you, though, to develop your own values about sex, because sex is one of the most powerful elements in our lives and, as I've tried to show, it can harm us if we play around with it. It's not for me to tell you what to do. I just want you to be more conscious of what you're doing.

Here are some sample questions:

> *Do I think there's a meaning to sex? If so, what is it? Or, to put it another way, what should having sex with someone **express**?*
> *What would make having sex with someone be right for me?*

*What would be some of the **wrong** reasons for having sex?*
How important is the sex part of a relationship to me? (Answer on a scale of 1-10)
Do I think sleeping around affects people spiritually, or inwardly?
Would it be better to wait until I'm married, or at least in a long-term committed relationship before I have sex?

Once you've worked out some basic values for sex I suggest you keep them somewhere private. Read them through from time to time. Change them as your understanding grows. Cherish them. The values that you work out for yourself about sex can help you in at least three ways. They can:

1. protect you from harm
2. help you feel good about yourself, and
3. help you have good relationships with the opposite sex.
   And
         that's
               no
                   small
                       thing.

Our next topic goes well beyond the personal.

The Law of Cosmic Balance

What's taken but not earned
must one day be returned

– E. W.

There's a deep law in life I call the law of cosmic balance. According to this law, if we hurt someone we have to redress this hurt. If we take more than we gave, we owe a debt which will have to be repaid. I believe this law holds true in all areas and in all relationships, although my sense of what's "earned" and what isn't, what's owing and what isn't, is considerably fuzzier than God's, or whoever it is keeping check on these matters.

For example, if we hurt someone's feelings and walk away from this hurting, walk across the car-park towards our car not bothering ourselves about it, then there's something left unresolved. If we're uncomfortable about this we may rationalize:

He/she asked for it.
I couldn't help it.
It wasn't my fault.
I don't have the time to er… "Hey yeh it's me are we still on for …"

It stays there, though, like an unpaid debt, like a broken promise. We may think we've got away with it, but the law of cosmic balance requires that eventually every debt has to be paid and balance has to be restored. I think unpaid debts, unresolved hurts, stay in our families and pass on to our descendants. Here's a story about this.

Years ago, one of my college students in LA – I'll call her Molly – told me after class one evening that she was going to kill herself. For some reason I took her seriously but, at the same time, didn't feel anxious. I asked her how she was planning on doing it. She said she was going to shoot herself in the head.

"Where?"

"In my car."

"Gonna be a bit messy isn't it? I mean, your blood all over the front seat and everything…Someone's got to clean it all up. I mean, like, gross. And, well, where will you hold the gun exactly? When you, you know, pull the trigger… It would be terrible to shoot yourself in the head but not die. People do that. Maybe spend the next 40 years as a vegetable…It would be a real bummer for your family. "

"Oh, I don't know Mr. Williams… " She was laughing and at the same time annoyed with me for making her laugh.

*The reason why she wanted to kill herself, she told me, was that everything she tried to do failed. She told me about all the seriously bad luck she'd been having, the jobs she'd lost through no fault of her own, getting her car stolen **three times in a month**, the sudden arrival of her domineering, non-English-speaking mother from Europe … it was terrible. I almost made the comment that wanting to kill herself had a certain logic to it. As she talked about her troubles I kept thinking this is it… it can't get any worse. And then it did. Reminded me of lines from one of my poems:*

"You think you've hit rock bottom
and it turns out to be a ledge
halfway down a precipice…"

She was a nice person. I couldn't understand why things were going so badly for her. I asked her about her grandparents and great grandparents. Turned out they were Mafia. Interesting, I thought. I said maybe she was paying back for some of the ways they'd taken from people, ripping them off, exploiting them.

"That's not fair."

"No, you're right Molly, it isn't," I said.

After a pause I said, very tentatively, "Maybe you tell God that you're willing to, well, make up for some of the stuff your ancestors did, but not all at once. Space it out a bit. I don't think God's all that strong on details, so let it be known that you need a break."

She looked skeptical.

"What have you got to lose Molly? Try it."

"Okay Mr. Williams," she sighed.

It worked. I met her six months later in a mall in Glendale, and she was okay. Hugs. Big smiles. Engagement ring.

The next story has a lot to do with our main subject.

Back in the old days, as I said earlier, I had quite a few relationships with women. Years later, after my time in Cilandak, when I was married and living in LA, I understood that in many of these affairs I had taken more than I had given. I'd sweep in with declarations of love, all quite sincere at the time but fading as the beloved was revealed as who she really was – a flawed human being with stale morning breath. As the magic died we'd quarrel or retreat into remoteness, and then I'd catch sight of another of those haunting faces and switch back to pursuit mode, leaving my partner behind.

I felt badly about what I could now see as the gap between what I gave and what I took. I thought of writing long letters to my old girlfriends asking their forgiveness, but had no idea where any of them were.

So I said, "Okay big G; as you may know, I'm a bit uneasy about the fact that I bedded a number of your female humans back over the years, and have the feeling I took more than I gave. You probably have a clearer idea of what the balance sheet says than I do.... but in case I'm right I'd like you to arrange things so that I can restore the balance. Whatever it takes. Before I die, preferably. If that's okay. Start when you like. I'm ready"

To my surprise, female students from my community college English classes started telling me about their experiences of being sexually abused by their fathers. I became a 'trusted male' to six of these girls. One of them was a big black girl named Sally, whom I often remember. From the age of three to thirteen she'd been through such horrific experiences of sexual abuse that I marveled at the fact that she was still sane and able to hold down a banking job and do college classes. Her father would take her to a pedophile house on Friday afternoon and pick her up – and his check – Sunday evening. One evening we were sitting, as usual, in the college cafeteria. Sally had been dredging up memories and telling them to me, often choking into silence as a particularly awful thing that some man had done to her came into consciousness.

"Then he.... then he....ahhh... "

"Go on. Go on Sally... "

"He... he....ahhh... "

"I'm here Sally."

"He held me by my wrists over the edge of the cliff and said if I ever told anyone he'd kill me... "

After an hour or so she sat back, sighed out a deep sigh, looked across the table at me and said, "Why do you sit there listening to this stuff?" The way things were between us I knew nothing but the truth would do.

"Well Sally," I said, "back in my past I took from women. Not in the way your father and all those other men took from you.... But I figured I'd taken more than I'd given, so I asked

God if I could give back to women and set the balance straight in the credit/debit columns. So... here I am listening to you talk about being hurt by men."

She thought, nodded and smiled. "Yeah. Okay. I can live with that," she said.

On another campus, at the end of an hour with a new class I was standing out on the balcony looking across at the sunlit mountains. One of my students – Daisy – asked me to check her writing for spelling mistakes. As I read I noticed drops of liquid falling on the page, which was odd, because it wasn't raining. Then I realized she was crying. I took her to a quiet corner in the cafeteria. She was in such a state she couldn't even talk at first, so to begin with I asked her questions and she nodded or shook her head. Most nights, I learnt, her dad came into her room saying he was looking for the dog. He'd do this pantomime of looking under the bed and between the sheets, and then he'd start doing stuff to her. Afterwards she'd cry for a long time. I told her that her first assignment was to put a lock on her door, photograph it, and bring me the photo. She did this, and got an A. After two or three similar meetings I talked to a counselor –with Daisy's permission – and soon, like the rest of "my girls", as I thought of them, Daisy was in a support group and undergoing individual therapy.

Eventually I moved back to England and lost touch with them. Maybe I helped them. I hope so. They certainly helped me, although I think Sally was the only one who knew how and why.

Sometimes people have talked to me about stuff they did that they regret doing:

"Yeah... I did some pretty stupid things back then..."

"I went crazy for a while. Slept with more people than I can remember."

" I was so pissed off when my parents got divorced I went totally wild just to show them.... even though they didn't know what I was doing and if they did they probably wouldn't have

cared. I was doing heroin, and I got pregnant and had an abortion, and I was gang-raped by a bunch of f....g bikers..."

" I first had sex when I was eleven. She was 13. I never looked back after that. I could get pretty well any girl I fancied to have sex with me. I always knew what to say. It's a kind of talent I guess. Then I.... I had this girl.... Crystal. She kind of fell in love with me. Got obsessed. She wouldn't stop bugging me. I got angry with her, told her to leave me alone. And she .... she nearly killed herself. Over me. Cut her wrists open. Over me! It really freaked me out."

Are there mistakes you feel remorseful or guilty about? If there are, and you want to restore the balance, here are some suggestions:

Note – these are not rules. You will not be graded.

Suggestion no. 1

Don't be heavy on yourself. Forgive yourself.

Suggestion no. 2:

Make an intention. Here's a general one: *'I sincerely intend to restore the balance in my life, to heal whatever I may have hurt or damaged, and to give back whatever I took. Please God make it possible for me to do this.'* Yours can be a lot more specific:

I intend to get back in touch with my father and ask his forgiveness, and make peace with him.

I intend to say Sorry to Sarah. I know I hurt her and I feel badly about this, and I really do want to make amends.

Giving back, restoring the balance, makes a lot more sense than going on guilt trips. If you took from people, look for ways to give back. You can always ask God – as I did – to help you find ways to restore the balance.

Cosmic Balance has a lot to do with our next topic.

ABORTION

Years after my abortion, I was married and became pregnant with my son. Carrying this baby was a painful reminder of my first child that never was allowed to live. But somehow, through this birth came reconciliation and resolution. –Renee (from "Project Rachel"
       – a recommended Catholic website.)

My concern is the spiritual aspect of abortion. Here's another story:

It was not long before I left England to go to Indonesia. Ann and I had been living together for about a year. We'd had a good time early on, but the relationship was going sour. Looking back, I see that I was a mess – needy and heavy. We were fighting a lot over silly little things. Ann got fed up with it and moved out of the apartment. I missed her. Kept calling her. Playing our favorite albums over the phone.

Eventually she came back and we carried on. Then it started to go bad again. Only this time she was pregnant.

Ann aborted the fetus. The baby.

It seemed like the best thing to do.

She told me she didn't want to see me any more.

Not for a long time.

That was one of the lowest points in my life. I loved kids, you see, and the abortion was, well, it was wrong.

Soon after this I went to Indonesia.

We wrote to one another for a while, then the letters got fewer and fewer, shorter and shorter. Occasionally I got news of her from friends. Once I went back to London and looked for her, without success. There was still something unresolved between us. I could feel it. Partly I was just really sorry that she'd known me at my worst. She was funny and smart and loving, and I realized we might have been happy if I'd had my act together. And partly it was the abortion. We'd killed the baby. Our baby. I kept thinking I should have said "NO Ann.... Let's have the baby and be its parents and get married and look after it." But I hadn't said that. I didn't really know anything about life, except how to love kids and help them learn and grow. Looking back from the other side of the world at what happened, I saw that, even though it was Ann's decision, I was at least 50% responsible, and I felt shame.

Seven years later I came home one evening to my house on the outskirts of Jakarta and found a note on my door.

"I'm in town, visiting my Dad. I'd like to see you. Please call the Hilton Hotel and ask for Rm. 363. Ann."

I drove into town and met her at the Hilton. We went to a restaurant by a lake. We talked and talked about our lives, about what we'd done, about how it had been since we last met. We forgave one another. We were pleased to find that we were still friends.

Before I took her back to her hotel she said, "There's one more thing...."

"Yes?"

"The abortion."

She looked away. There were tears in her eyes.

"It was awful, afterwards. You came over here and left me with .... the whole mess. I was really f....ed up. I hated you. I

was angry with you for a long time. I'm not angry any more, but there's still a shadow there. The baby. Our baby..."

She cried.

I put my arms around her.

I was crying too. We had both been carrying this regret, this shame, all that time.

Next day I took Ann to a small craft enterprise I'd set up. Indonesian workers making lamps and lampshades. As we walked around we found Sri, a smart young women in her early twenties who supervised some of the workers, sitting alone looking very upset.

She told me she was pregnant, and that her husband had just lost his job caddying on the big Western golf course in Jakarta, so they didn't have enough money for the baby. I knew that, in the Javanese way, they had several relatives living with them, and that things had been tight.

Ann and I went off to talk. We decided to set up a bank account for Sri. We each put in $500 – a big sum of money for Sri. I spoke to the bank manager, told him about Sri, and asked him to look out for her.

Then we drove back to the factory and told Sri what we had done, that she could have her baby. She was ecstatic.

Ann left for England the next day. When we said goodbye at the airport it felt as though the shadow had been lifted.

This was my earliest experience of the law of balance – the principle that if you take something away, you have to put something back. Ann and I had aborted a baby. We owed the universe a life. Maybe because we both sincerely regretted this act we were given the chance to enable a child to be born, a life to be lived, and thus take care of the debt.

I'm certain that abortion, like sexual intercourse, is a lot more complex and profound than the physical act we may consider it to be. I came across a gut-wrenching article on a website: Abortionfacts.com, entitled 'When the doll breaks' by Theresa Karminski Burke. The article's too long to reproduce here; it tells the story of a girl named Marita who became cynical and depressed following an abortion. The main event in the article is a game called 'Baby Soccer', in which people at a dorm party have a few beers and then kick the heads of decapitated dolls around the room. The game gets more and more violent, with people gouging out dolls' eyes and burning their faces and thighs with cigarettes.

"Like Marita", says the writer, *"many of the young women and men drawn into this game had also lost children to abortion. 'Baby soccer' provided a symbolic means to mock, belittle and display mastery over the babies who were never allowed to be born but who still haunted their memories."*

Would this pattern of sick acting – out be broken if those responsible for aborting babies acknowledged what they had done, and maybe participated in a different sort of ritual, as suggested later in this section? There are never any guarantees, of course, but I would say: "Very probably."

My wife Amelia told me this story:

A couple I know had an abortion. The business they'd been developing was failing, and they were heavily in debt. They felt they simply couldn't afford another child.

They told me about the abortion.

Soon afterwards I had a dream that related to it.

In the dream a young child – a blond boy – came to me. I saw that he had a big gash, a hole on top of his head, on the crown. I understood in the dream that he'd been spiritually injured. The wound on his head was where his connection with God should be.

He said, "I've been hurt, and my parents don't know it." He obviously came to me to say this. I felt in the dream that he was asking for help from me. I woke up and immediately began praying for him. I felt that was what he needed me to do.

Our culture doesn't pay much attention to the human or spiritual significance of the big experiences: sex, pregnancy, marriage, work, parenting, old age, death. Maybe some girls or women who are pregnant feel or *know* that this life growing in their body has a soul but don't talk about it, partly because of their culture, and partly because the people around them – boyfriend, husband, parents, counselors – may be urging them to have an abortion, and don't want to hear about this.

I can't imagine how hard it must be to find that you're pregnant and you're only thirteen, and your parents are treating you like you're a whore. Or, you're married and are overjoyed to discover that you're pregnant and then your husband says that if you have the baby he'll leave you. Under such circumstances it must be very difficult to make a clear, deeply felt decision. Go one way and maybe you have a baby at a time when it's difficult for you to take care of him or her. Go the other way and maybe you'll have the clear feeling that you're destroying a life. Then you have to choose the lesser of two harms. Which choice that may be is up to you.

But please remember this: having an abortion *isn't the end of the world.* If we took then we can give back. If we hurt or injured then we can heal. If we destroyed then we can create.

I don't believe we can do this alone however. Or, let me put it this way: I think it's easier if we ask for help from a power that's higher than ourselves. If you can believe in this or, if not believe, than at least to accept it as a possibility, then I recommend that you reach out to this power for help. A young woman told me she thinks the Virgin Mary takes care of the souls of aborted children.

Between one quarter and one third of all babies conceived in America are aborted. According to researcher Dr. Anne Speckham, of the University of Minnesota, about one in three women who have abortions have an experience in which they 'perceive visitations with their child.' [1]

That's about half a million women a year apparently having some experience of the spirit or presence of their aborted child. Maybe some of them are imagining the baby being there – creating a kind of 'phantom child' through the intensity of their feeling. And maybe some of them really are being contacted by the spirit of the child they might have had.

Here's an account of an abortion experience written by an old friend:

I was 23 years old and attending Art School in England in the late 60s. I was living in a shared house which was the meeting place for lots of students as well as "townies" and a drug hangout. Neurotic and insecure as I was, getting pregnant by my boyfriend was not on my agenda. It seems unreal now, but the social message at that time was "Well, if you get pregnant, you have an abortion."…simple as that.

The "Relate" agency had just opened up in London. This was an anti-establishment, social project that helped young people on drugs, as well as desperate young girls, needing safe abortions. At that time, thousands of girls were coming over to England to terminate unwanted pregnancies, and as I walked the grey rainy London streets, looking for the Relate offices, I felt a sudden kinship with all these desperate girls and women that seemed to stretch back through the ages…..the disgrace… the sometimes lethal backstreet abortions….the general misery. We didn't seem to have come very far, except that now at least there was some degree of safety.

It was all set up and I duly arrived at the "Clinic". I put that word in quotes because it was a horrible long room full of

*camp beds only six inches apart and the "operating theatre",
just a little room off to the side. Only two proper hospital beds
were in evidence, and it seemed to all of us that they were stuffing
in as many girls as they could each day. It was a factory. We
each in turn had to sit at a desk in full view and hearing of
everyone and give our reasons for needing a termination. We
were then led one by one into the other room and then walked
back in between two orderlies who hadn't even bothered to wash
the blood off their aprons!*

*When my turn came, I asked the nurse to hold my hand...
then I went under the anesthetic.*

*Suddenly, I "saw" the baby...a huge disc of light and I knew
in that instant that what I had done was wrong for me.....
BUT...in the same moment, I understood that the "baby" was
not just a collection of cells but a fully human soul...enormous
in its beingness, and with this knowledge a total awareness of
the existence if God. It was an undeniably real sensation – a
blinding flash. Simultaneously, behind the baby, I saw another
disc of light, which I knew to be an angel, and from this being
emanated TOTAL forgiveness.*

*I came out of the anesthetic crying and saying "Oh God...
what have I done? My poor baby." I was told to shut up as I
was upsetting the other girls.*

From that moment, my spiritual search began.

*I will always carry that experience with me. Nowadays, I
find it impossible to pass any judgment on anyone facing that
same situation. I pray that the parents might not go through
with it for their sake but it's a sacred space between them and
God. I sometimes feel for the men involved...they seem to have
very little power in this area. It's true that the woman has to
cope with the physical and emotional consequences but I feel
men also suffer a sense of loss. How wonderful it would be
if every single child who came to this earth, was welcomed,
wanted and loved.*

I'm not trying to *prove* anything here. And since I've been at least partially responsible for an abortion, I'm certainly in no position to judge anyone. But I'm certain that there are spiritual consequences to abortion. A fetus is a life. If we destroy the physical body of that life we must face the possibility that there is a being, a soul that has been cast into a limbo by the abortion. He or she may be stuck. It is our responsibility to free this stuck, trapped soul so that he or she can go on. If we don't, then it is likely that this soul will suffer, and that it will become part of our psychic burden, or karma.... whatever you want to call it.

Here's a story that Matthew, an old friend, told me.

Years ago I was in love with a girl called Maria. We went away for a weekend in the Lassen area of North California. It was winter and there was snow in the mountains. Everywhere it was white and quiet. We were staying in a cabin that belonged to some friends of mine. We came back from a day in the snow....both wet and cold but feeling great. I lit a log fire and we jumped into bed and watched the firelight on the walls. I asked her to marry me and she said Yes. We made love. That was one of the best times of my life.

Time passed. We were back in our lives. She came to see me one night. Told me she was pregnant. I was so happy. I kept grinning and saying 'Allelujah!' Not that I'm religious, but it seemed like a good word at the time.

Then she began to close up. I could feel her retreating from me. From us. She said she needed time to think. I didn't know what was going on. I couldn't get through to her. It was bizarre. Here we were, in love, almost engaged, having a baby.... and she was, I don't know, she was off somewhere.

One afternoon I was in the University library working on my Master's thesis, and I suddenly felt this terrible wrenching pain in my guts. I fell to the floor whimpering and retching, clutching at my belly. Someone came and helped me up, asked me if I was okay. After a while the worst of it passed. On my way home I suddenly knew what was going on. Maria had had an abortion. Later I found out it happened right at the time I was experiencing those symptoms in the University Library.

I drove to her house. She was out. I sat in my car and waited. Later that evening she came home. A girlfriend helped her out of her car and walked her to her front door. I got out of my car and stood there, watching. She looked across at me, then turned and went in.

It took me a long time to forgive her. I had to do my own abortion. I had to kill the love I felt for her.

Later that year, in the summer, I drove back to the cabin in Lassen. I sat there for a long time. I cried for a while. I wanted to say how sorry I was to the baby. I said, "I don't know who you are. I don't know if you're a little boy or a little girl. I'm sorry for what happened. I love you. Maybe one day you'll want to try again. I would like to be your daddy".

I made a figurine out of pine needles and tiny cones. I put it in the fireplace and set light to it. I asked that the baby's soul be taken home. I didn't know what I was doing. It felt right to do what I did, that's all. I was thinking of the smoke rising into the clean mountain air and disappearing into the sky.

Whether there's a soul or spirit or some kind of non-physical presence that survives the destruction of its body is a question with no clear answer, unless you've had the kind of experience Kathy describes in this account:

I was young. In my early twenties. I didn't know then what I know now. I wasn't married. Had a relationship that I knew wasn't going to work out. Anyway, I got pregnant and had an abortion.

Later, much later, I realized I'd made a mistake. I felt I'd done something that was, well, wrong. I had a lot of regrets in me. About the abortion, I mean. I wasn't a church-goer or anything, but I believed – still do – in God. Or, in something that was higher and more powerful than me. This belief became the center of my life.

So I prayed – or asked – to be forgiven. It felt like the prayer went very deep.

Afterwards I felt better. Things lightened up.

Many years later I married and had a baby. About a year after her birth I felt a presence and began to sense there was still something unresolved.

I didn't know what to do, so I talked to some friends about it. One of them was an intuitive, a psychic; she could kind of feel things psychically.

She said the soul of the child I'd aborted had not yet been committed, had not 'gone over', as she said, completely.

So we agreed to do a group prayer for the child, to help it on its way.

I had an incredible experience. This is what happened:

I met the child. It was a girl. (I'd thought it was a boy.) She was wise. She said to me:

"I agreed to stay with you until your own child was born. But you've forgotten that agreement, and now it's time for you to let me go." (At that time my daughter was one year old.)

So then what happened was that I held the aborted child in my arms. I was taken to a dimension I'd never seen before or since. I was allowed to accompany her on her journey up to a certain point. Then the line stopped for me. I didn't see anyone there to welcome and accept her, but I felt I was releasing her to continue her journey to where she was supposed to be.

I felt that her soul's progress had been interrupted, but because, after the abortion, I'd become committed to my own spiritual path or progress, she'd been protected and was able to return to where she was supposed to be. But I knew that it was only because I'd begun to come to life inwardly that I was able to release her in this way.

If you or your partner have had an abortion then it may be hard for you to confront the possibility that the being whose body was destroyed is still, in some way, in some dimension, alive. You may well have gone through a lot of pain and upset already, and now I'm suggesting that maybe it's not over yet, that maybe there's more to be considered, there's more to be done. Perhaps you're feeling so down about losing your baby that you just want to put the whole thing behind you, forget it, bury it, get on with your life.

Here's Amelia again:

I hadn't seen or spoken with Maggie for more than 2 years.

One night I had a powerful dream about her. I dreamt that she was very sick, and dying, and was asking for help.

After the dream I woke up and had to get out of bed and pray for her. I had no choice in the matter.

The feeling that she was sick and desperate went on. I was very worried about her. So after a while I got in touch with her.

She said she was fine physically, but was in a terrible state emotionally – depressed, suffering, even suicidal. She said she'd had an abortion (agreed to by her husband) and she hadn't told anyone about it, even her friends in the local church she attended. She said that because of the abortion she felt too ashamed or unworthy to reach out and ask for help from the church she attended, and she felt cut off from grace.

She said that by my writing to her, her faith was restored, and that even if she'd made a mistake she could go back to church and gain the support she needed. And more importantly she now felt she had the right to turn to God, and that God hadn't turned away from her.

If you've had an abortion, dear reader, you need to heal. You need to become whole again. You need to forgive yourself and love yourself. Also, I believe, you need to take care of the soul of the baby who came to you.

There are three dimensions in post-abortion healing:

1. Physical.

Among the possible physical consequences of abortion are: sterility, incontinence, tubular pregnancies, infection and a greater likelihood of future miscarriages.
(See the website <abortionfacts.com> for a full discussion of these medical consequences.)

2. Emotional.

Among the possible psychological consequences of abortion are:
depression, suicidal thoughts/attempts (research shows that women who had an abortion are twice as likely to commit suicide as women who gave birth), increase in self-destructive activities – drugs, alcohol, eating disorders and promiscuity; outbreaks of anger; problems at school or at work. A really excellent source of advice and support can be found at:: <afterabortion. org>. especially their 'Individual recovery steps' section. See also the touching website: <Abortionwarmemorial.org>

3. Spiritual.

(I think the spiritual consequences apply to both partners).

How do you heal spiritually from an abortion? If you belong to a religion, ask for help. You might ask for prayers to be said for yourself and for the child you lost. You might find powerful guidance in Dr. Kenneth McCall's book "Healing the Family Tree".

If you're not religious this doesn't mean that you're not able to reach God, or talk to God, or pray to God. God, after all, is not religious. If you're the father or the mother of an aborted child you can pray. Here are some prayers I wrote that you might find appropriate. Feel free to ignore them, change them, or combine them.... They're written for one person, but can easily be adapted for two people.

1.

Little one
my little child
my baby
please forgive me.
You came to me for life
and I turned you away.
Know that I love you, little one
and I know that I am deeply sorry.
Again, I ask your forgiveness
and I pray that you may be free
to journey on
and find your home

2.

Oh source of all life
where I took
may I be allowed to give
where I wounded
may I be allowed to heal
where I destroyed
may I be allowed to create
where I did wrong
may I be guided to do what is right
may I be forgiven.

3.
Almighty God
creator of all beings
I have taken the life
of an innocent child
and I am truly sorry.
I bow down my head in shame and regret
I pray that the shadow of this deed
be taken from me
now and forever.
I pray for forgiveness.
Almighty God
may your angels enfold
and bring into light
the soul of this child.

You can put things together and make up your own short simple ritual, with the purpose of freeing the aborted child so that he or she can go on, and for you to seek forgiveness both from the child and from God.

You need a quiet place. No phones, no interruptions. Make it special.

You might have something that represents the child – a flower or a doll you made (like my friend Dave) or tiny bootees. Something like that. Candles. Music. (Adagio, by Samuel Barber, is a deeply consoling piece of music. Or the Tallis Fantasia by Vaughn Williams. Or a slow song by the Celtic group Clannad.) Prayers. Invite people you think would be in tune with what you're doing.

Once you've completed the ritual, recognize that you've made your act of repentance, and *don't let yourself feel bad about what you did any more.*

Let go of it.

Here's a quote from an extraordinary book:

Abortion…. is contrary to that which is natural. The spirit coming into the body feels a sense of rejection and sorrow. It knows that the body was to be his, whether it was conceived out of wedlock or was handicapped or was only strong enough to live a few hours. But the spirit also feels compassion for the mother, knowing that she made a decision based on the knowledge she had. [2]

Ideally, you go through this healing as a couple. If, as often happens, the man makes it clear that he's not going to stay around then the girl, or woman, has to go through the healing without him. If this is your situation, then whatever happens to the man is between him and God. Don't burden yourself with anger towards him.

If you're pregnant, I suggest you seriously consider having the baby. In one website I read a very moving letter written by a girl whose mother was raped and became pregnant. The girl is so grateful to her mother *for letting her live.*

If it is truly wrong for the baby to be born, then there's the possibility that the mother will have a miscarriage. My first marriage was a total disaster; my wife and I fought every day. She became pregnant. We still went on fighting. A month or so later she had a miscarriage. I think our baby decided – wisely – this was not a good time to be born, and returned to where he or she had come from.

To sum up this section: I believe abortion has spiritual consequences. However, let me say it again: *It's not the end of the world.*

I believe it's up to us to face these consequences, and to:

a. Help the aborted child to proceed on its spiritual journey, and

b. seek ways to be healed ourselves.

Of the two, I believe the second is the most essential. I have the feeling – based on conversations with a number of women who've had abortions, and on my own sense of spiritual laws – that the souls of aborted children are somehow taken care of. Sometimes however, as we have seen, they need some help from us.

CELIBACY

The fuller levels of feeling, the deep levels of tenderness and intimacy, can easily be lost because sexual activity is so dominating and tends to hold the focus of attention when people are making love. You may long to express these deeper parts to your lover but may end up expressing only the sexual.

- Gabrielle Brown

During most of my early years in Cilandak I was celibate. At first this was a matter of circumstance; there was relatively little opportunity to be sexually active, but soon I made the conscious decision to go celibate and asked Big G. to help me remain chaste for as long as was needed. And not a day longer please. I had the feeling that it would be good for me. I wasn't sure why, but in that early Cilandak period there was very little that I was sure about, except that – mostly quite innocently – I'd done a lot of things that weren't good for me, and had been given the chance to put things right. I had come to a place where this could happen and, I realized, I was incredibly lucky. Slowly, so slowly and subtly that I didn't notice it happening, I was being relieved of the cargo of my past mistakes.

The decision to be celibate was easier over there because, as I said, Javanese culture was less overtly sexualized. (Java is a Moslem country, and I think Islam is a lot more straightforward about sex than Christianity. In fact, I've heard it said that whereas Jesus made it possible for us to be redeemed during our lifetimes, thereby freeing us from the great wheel of reincarnation, Mohammed made it possible for human beings to worship the Almighty while making love. But I digress.)

I realized that this cleansing process would take a lot longer if I thought of myself as a passive entity waiting to be cured by the great MD in the sky. I could help this process along by being as vigilant a gatekeeper to my inner as possible. If I found myself recalling a steamy scene from the past I'd interrupt the sequence with a good-humored bustling intrusion:

"Well we all know what happens next so, I tell you what, let's er let's stop the movie right there shall we and take ourselves off for a nice long walk, okay? Or maybe even a long cold shower...? Sorry about this but that's the way it is."

Not long after I made my intention, my maid Samiam took some time off to have a baby and was replaced by new maid named Ida. Ida was very pretty and vivacious, flirtatious even, and she dressed provocatively. Back from school one afternoon I found myself looking down the front of her dress and hearing the primal growl deep in my guts, and I thought, " *This could get very messy.*" I asked her to sit down, then, slowly and with much searching through my English-Indonesian dictionary, I told her she must dress more modestly while she was working for me. When she finally understood what I was saying she looked very confused and embarrassed –"malu" in Indonesian – and was near to tears. I told her she could go home, and I'd see her tomorrow.

"*Thanks for the test, big G.,*" I said that evening. There was no answer. Apparently the deity does not respond to irony. The primrose path man, still very much alive in me, was infuriated by my act of self-denial. "*I can't believe you did that man... I mean what is your PROBLEM?*" The white wall man, still unsure as to where all this was going, seemed encouraged.

The word celibacy may evoke images of monks or priests living in a lifelong state of chastity, or of puritans or fundamentalists heatedly denouncing the sins of the flesh. But I've met people for whom celibacy seemed to be a natural unforced state. Some years ago Salamah and I facilitated a discussion group for young people called 'Sex before Marriage.' It was a very frank, open exchange in which people talked about their experiences of sex, their feelings about it and their understandings. One of the participants, an attractive 25 year-old Austrian woman named Hilde, told us she was a virgin. I think she was a high BLOB person. She said she wasn't against sex, and it wasn't a matter of "sin" or anything like that; she simply hadn't met the right man, the man she could make love with. She said she'd met many men she'd liked, and been attracted to some, but a voice inside her always told her to wait, that this wasn't the man she should give herself to. She said she wasn't anxious or frustrated about this. When she met the right man she'd know. But first they'd get married, and then they'd complete their union, they'd make love for the first time.

I was touched by her story and wrote this monolog:

The diamond
I used to think there was something wrong with me
something missing, like an energy that's alive and real
in the lives of everyone I know, that's all around me
in films and books and magazines , songs, conversations...
Sometimes I meet someone
at a party or, you know, just doing what I do
and I feel an attraction
like a warm buzz in the pit of my stomach
and I think 'I like him.'
But then he says something that feels ... not wrong exactly
it just jars me. Could be the way he looks at me
or smiles or walks
it shows me something about him that I didn't see before
and I think 'No he's not the one.'
and the door in my heart that opened to him closes
and the feeling of being attracted dies.
Sometimes it's hard when a guy wants me
and I say 'I like you but not in that way.'
They always take it as a rejection.
I wish they didn't.
I don't know how you can want someone who doesn't want
you.
It doesn't make sense to me.
I think, if the feeling's right between two people
then they'll always want each other at the same time.
It won't be: 'I want to go to bed with you and I know you
don't want to
but come and sit here and have another glass of wine and ....'
It'll be.... it'll be....it won't be like that.
Sometimes I think I'm being protected.
A sort of spiritual chastity belt.
I'm glad really.

There was a guy I met. I wanted him.
When we talked there was this feeling we could say anything
we could say things we didn't even know we were going to say.
We talked for six hours in a coffee bar
then we went and sat on the grass
on a little hill on the edge of town
and suddenly it was there
and I knew he was feeling it too.
I sat there with my eyes closed, waiting.
He held my hand. It was the first time we'd touched.
I thought, if he strokes the skin on the palm of my hand
and the insides of my fingers
I will melt, like honey, and trickle down the hill.
He said 'It's not the right time. Is it?'
I said No. Or I thought it and he heard me.
He said 'If God gives you a diamond
and you say Thank you and give it back
God will give you a bigger diamond.'
So.....
I'm not waiting for him.
I'm waiting for what I felt when I was with him.
I think that's why I met him.

If you settle for second best
that's what you get.

The decision I made to go celibate when I was in Cilandak was easier because I wasn't seeing anyone. Going celibate as a couple is obviously more difficult. There's an episode from my past I still remember with some regret:

I was on a teacher training course, and I met a woman called Louise. We started going out, and soon we were sleeping with one another. One evening we were out for a walk on Hampstead Heath, a big park in North London, and she turned to me and said, " I really like you. I'm not in love with you, but I like being with you, and I want to go on being with you. And I don't want to hurt your feelings or anything…. but I think we should stop sleeping with one another for a while. I can't explain it… I just…. I mean, it's not that I don't like sleeping with you. I do. In a way sex between us is too good. I just want to … clear the space a bit. Is that okay?"

I wasn't mature enough for this option. I said Yes … good idea… I can live with that… But I felt rejected. I pretended to go along with the new regime, but I wanted her to want me again. I kind of glimpsed the way it could be, but, without admitting it to myself, I wanted to be the one who made the decisions. I kept trying to seduce her. "I just feel so much for you, and I want you…" I had this plan of warming her up, as it were, then saying, "No, we shouldn't be doing this," so that I could be the one in control. Stupid idiot. Louise knew what was going on. She didn't accuse me or blame me. She just said goodbye. Which was a great pity, because I really liked being with her.

I think we can tell if there's too much sex in a relationship. What's too much? There are no objectively established limits. It depends on the quality or content of the partners' union. If every touch, every movement, every sound, every give and take expresses deep love for the other, and if the partners are intent upon and fully aware of what pleases the other, then the love-making will be greatly more satisfying and complete than mere physical coupling. Quality rather than quantity. Someone told me the other day that the man should aim at giving the woman five – yes that's 5 – orgasms.

When partners are having a lot of sex they lose touch with the other elements and feelings that are potentially alive between them. I can name some of these elements – tenderness, delight in little things, an intimacy based on both sexual awareness and a different, more companionable feeling – but they have to be experienced to be known. Louise wanted us to be free of the rather heavy sexual vibe so that we could find out more about one another than whatever we discovered in bed.

Years ago in L.A. I knew a couple: Colin and Melissa, who'd been married about nine years and had a three year-old daughter – Anita. I thought of them as the ideal couple. He was handsome; she was beautiful. They got on well together. They both liked sports. She was a successful children's book writer; he was a tenured English instructor in one of the colleges I taught at.

One evening Colin told me something that astonished me. He said for more than four years after Anita was born Melissa felt no desire for him. She said she still loved him as much as she ever had, but her libido had simply vanished.

"It was hell, especially at first," he said. "I don't know how many times I jumped out of bed late at night, feeling horny and totally frustrated. Threw some clothes on, drove away to a bar, or some remote place where I could yell at the stars."

They tried counseling, prescription drugs, acupuncture, herbal remedies, soft porn ... nothing worked. She'd cry and say how sorry she was, and how much she loved him, and ask him to hold her. She asked him to be patient, to wait, to stay close to her, not to leave her. Sometimes he thought he'd go off and start an affair with another woman so that Melissa would be jealous and maybe make love again, just to keep him.

"Even if that had worked, it would have felt wrong. I'd be using someone else."

After nearly three years of this he finally reached a kind of resolution. He decided to try to accept the marriage on her terms.

"I couldn't leave her. I just couldn't do it. And I just couldn't sleep with someone else. But if I stayed… well… I knew if we went on fighting about sex it wouldn't work. I guess she couldn't pretend to want to have sex with me. And the more frustrated and angry I got, the worse she felt, and that made her tighten up even more. So…that was the situation. I mean it was ridiculous. I couldn't believe it was happening to me. To us, I should say.

I don't know how I managed it, but one night I said, 'Okay Melissa. Let's just love one another, look after Anita, and have a home and a life together, and, and not have sex. Not bother about it. Maybe one day it will come back.'

The way I figured it … whenever I tried to touch her, or, you know, tried to arouse her, she rejected me. And this bummed me out. And then I'd get angry because I was bummed out, and that made her feel more guilty So the way to avoid feeling bummed out was to avoid being rejected.

And the way to avoid being rejected was **to wait for her to come to me!**

How about that?

How about that? I mean, Gahd……..

Did I **know** that one day she'd come to me?

No I didn't. I just hoped she would.

Wasn't easy. I was out one day with a fishing buddy and I caught a 20 pound salmon. Put up a hell of a fight. We got it in the boat and Jim said, 'Good as sex, isn't it?' I laughed, 'Right!' Just a casual remark. but there was this kind of wince inside me. Guys talk about it all the time. And there I was, a married freaking monk…

But I did it. Don't know how. I could cuddle up to Melissa, put my arms round he, and it was okay, you know. And I'd feel so tender. Sure I got horny. She's…wow… Some nights I'd have to force myself to think about other stuff. Like I'd think about a lake in the high Sierras… we went camping there one summer, before we were married. It was when I knew I really loved *her, that this was it. I'd go for a swim every morning, jump right in off a rock. Jeez it was cold. Nut -freezer. I'd remember that.*

I still have no idea why it happened. I mean, why Melissa lost her libido for so long. Then one night she turned towards me, reached out and touched my face. She said, "Thank you for waiting."

She kissed me.

And we made love.

It was… It was incredible. Like nothing I've ever experienced. Out of this world.

Jeez, I love her. I love her so much. I never knew it could be like this. And, you know what I found out? I found out that we still loved one another even though we weren't making love. And that… that's really something."

Last story, this from a young woman I'll call Lisa:

I was involved with this guy, Ivan. He was a total jerk. I didn't know this at first. It was when he moved in with me… it turned out he was incredibly jealous. Asking me who I was talking to on the phone. Turning up at my work with some lie about he'd locked himself out and could he borrow my keys, but really there just to check out the guys who worked there. Not wanting me to go out with my friends. It was scary. My girlfriends all said he'd get violent if I stayed around, so I left him. Got a job in Sacramento.

Anyway, this was a lot later, I'd forgotten about him… I was driving down to LA to see my mom. I stopped off at a diner for a break, and there was this strange thing happened. I was walking across the car park when I suddenly felt like this big weight was being lifted off me, lifted from my chest and shoulders. I felt so light I thought I was going to levitate. Felt like I could breathe again, really breathe for the first time in ages. And I knew, I don't know how but I knew it was Ivan, leaving me. He was being lifted out of me… the feeling of him that had been there all the time and I hadn't even known. Three years since I'd left him. It was kind of spooky in a way, but I tell you, wow, it felt great to be free of him at last.

Yeeeee…

The other thing I … now I was ready for a man. I was ready to love again.

Three years of celibacy to be free of the effects of a relationship. That was what Lisa needed, and, looking back, that was roughly how long I needed in Cilandak. Not that – to say it again – there are objective measures in this area. If you were to ask me: "Emmanuel, how long does it take to get over, really get over, a relationship?" I'd have to say, "It depends." It probably takes longer than most of us think. But there are so many variables: how long did the relationship last? How important was the sexual element? (Or, to put it baldly, how often did the partners have sex?) Were they living together? (The more intimate the relationship the longer it takes to get over it, and living together obviously deepens and intensifies the intimacy.)

What did I regain during those long hot days sitting by the wall? Not my purity. I learnt a lot of truths about myself as I looked back at my experiences as a primrose path man, and even though – as I discovered – I can be freed of the effects of the experiences that taught me these truths I don't unlearn the truths themselves. We can't go backwards. Neither innocence nor purity can be fully regained, but what you arrive at, sooner or later, is something bigger, which I'd call integrity.

I like this comment about going celibate from Miguel (whom I quoted earlier):

For me, it wasn't about reclaiming purity, at least not at first. It was about getting clarity of motivation. I realized that my sex desires, when followed, didn't leave me feeling like I understood things. I needed time to press reset and get more control.

Going celibate for a while can be a good thing, but it can be very hard. Awakened by our consumerist culture, voices inside us squawk like fledglings in a nest: "I want this I want that give me this give me that…" We are continually urged to get what we want without stopping to think about whether we need it, or even really want it. So the notion of going celibate seems both counter-cultural, and counter to some rather strong biological drives. Plus, if we're in a relationship, it may not be what our partner wants. So the decision to opt for a period of celibacy has to be made carefully. I don't like to give advice, but here are some suggestions:

1. Know why.

List the reasons why you want to go celibate. You might include:

* facts about the danger of sexually transmitted diseases,
* how you think sleeping around may have affected you,
* how you think going celibate might benefit you.

2. Make your intention.

Your intention is a promise you make to yourself. Keep it explicit and realistic. I suggest you think about your intention, write it down, then create your own "vowing ritual." Rituals are the outer expression of an inner wish, or movement, and can be a source of personal strength and guidance. They're a way for you to tell yourself: "I really mean this."

Your intention might look something like this:

"I ... (your name) intend to go without sex for...............
so that my relationship with Tanya/ Michael may be made
lighter and more loving/ so that I may be more aware of the
nature of my sexual feelings, and more in control of them."

After 'for.... ' you'd put the length of time you think
you can manage. "48 hours.,...." " a week.... " "Three
years.... " I recommend against vague phrases like "for
as long as I am able..." The inner self needs things to
be clear. The servants need to know what's going on; it's
the boss's job to tell them.

You might complete your intention with a prayer to
a higher power in which you ask for help. You can do
this even if you have no faith in the possibility of there
being any higher power. What have you got to lose? As
the French philosopher Pascal wrote: *Let us weigh the*
gain and the loss in wagering that God is. Let us estimate these
two chances. If you gain, you gain all; if you lose, you lose
nothing. Wager, then, without hesitation that He is.

So your complete intention might go something like
this:

"I, Ribald Farthingale, intend to abstain from sex for three
months. I ask that God (Christ, the great spirit, my spirit, the
angels etc) may help me carry out this intention, so that I may
come closer to my true self and closer to my creator." Or words
to that effect.

Be honest with yourself. If you make an intention
like this, know what you mean by *"abstain from sex."*
Obviously this includes intercourse. But what about oral
sex? Know where your line is. The servants need clear
parameters.

If you've been very active sexually, then you should
seriously consider abstaining from all sexual contact.
I'll repeat that: *If you've been very active sexually, then you*
should seriously consider abstaining from all sexual contact.

It gets easier. You will find yourself becoming clearer and lighter and more radiant and happier. No no no turns into yes yes yes, oh YES!

3. Making it work

Read your intention (aloud, if possible) every night before you go to sleep, and every morning before you start your day. Please, stay light. If you blow it, forgive yourself and start again. Hold the intention there, inside you. If you make it through a month, great.

Addictions and habits can be hard to break. The energies in us that get off on sleeping around won't give up without a struggle. They'll try to derail us, because they don't want us to succeed.

You may be in a relationship that's feeling unbalanced. You may think that sex has become too important, that it's taking precedence over everything else. Maybe you have a fight, for example, and you're shouting at one another, hurting each other... and then, with the anger still smoldering, you have sex. Or you may be sexually obsessed, always touching, not in a light loving way, but sexily, stroking one another in crowded places, feeling one another in cinemas or cars or wherever... looking for that tense hot look in your partner's eyes which tells you he/she is feeling aroused, and wants to have sex with you, SOON.... NOW!

If it's like this then maybe you both need to cool it for a while.

Easy for me to say, I know. When you're in the grip of obsessive sexual desire *it's really hard to stop*. You have a battle on your hands. Fight to return the ruler to the throne. If you can accept the possibility of a higher power – then pray to that power for help. Pray deeply and sincerely for this force in you to be lifted from you, to be taken away. Create a cleansing dance, maybe with some friends. Paint a picture of it on a big sheet of paper – jagged blacks and orange, slashes of hot red – and, when it's dry, burn it. There's lots of space up there.

If you're sexually obsessed by someone, then you are, I believe, suffering from an illness, just as the alcoholic is, or the drug addict. You are addicted. You're at serious risk of losing dignity and self-respect. If this is your situation, check out Sexaholics Anonymous on the web. They can help. And there's information about abstinence and related topics, on: www.plannedparenthood.org.

Making Babies

The importance of the quality of our state at the moment of conception seems to me to be fundamental to the future of the world over the next few generations. … If humankind's attitude towards this important insight can be changed, the future of humankind could be very different and peace could come to the world.

– Arthur Abdullah Pope

The main theme of this book is that there's a spiritual aspect to sex. This is not a truth you'll find "on the street" or discussed in the media. It's not a truth that can be proved, although there's quite a lot of anecdotal evidence around that supports it. If it is true – if, indeed, there is a spiritual aspect to sex – what difference does it make? It's up to each one of us how we answer this question.

I've tried to show that there are spiritual consequences to having sex – that it's never casual, however casually we treat it. I hope that readers of this book will be able to make more conscious choices about sex.

Great blessings may come our way if and when our sex lives come more in line with our higher human selves. We may experience the true meaning of bliss – as in the waves of light, the angelic throng, the sky-high infusions… An even greater and more lasting blessing is that when we make love in a worshipful, loving way *we may become parents of children who have noble characters and high souls.*

Different babies have different basic levels of being. If they were all the same, human beings would be a lot less varied in their basic levels of being. There are babies with low BLOBS and babies with high BLOBs. The latter tend to become adults with high BLOBs, and high BLOB adults are good for the world, bringing out the best in everyone they meet. So the question arises: How do we make babies with high levels of being?

When the man and woman conceive a child, the content of their love-making determines the content of that child. This means that our inner states are tremendously important when we make love. The quality of the partners' inner feelings act as a kind of lens that attracts a higher or lower soul. If they've had a fight that evening, or if one of them watched a horror or pornographic movie before going to bed, or is disturbed by something bad that happened at work, these feelings will be in the sperm (just as nicotine will be there if he's a smoker, and alcohol if she's a drinker, and so on) or the mother's egg, and enter and influence the inner nature of the child.

Everything is connected to everything else.

As I said before, there are no walled-off compartments in our psyches. An English friend told me that he'd experienced the inner feelings of his parents when he was conceived. He said his father was sexually very dominating and aggressive, while his mother was unresponsive and submissive – "Lie there and think of England." He said he recognized these two states as typical patterns in his behavior *throughout his adult life.*

When we come together cleanly and worshipfully then not only will our love-making be more blissful than we ever thought possible, but also, if we conceive a child, then he or she will be a real blessing to us and the world.

So everything is present when we have sex. Every part of us. Not just our bodies, not just our feelings, but also our spirits, or if you prefer, our deeper selves. As the following quote shows, this isn't such a strange idea:

… for many Americans sex is not just moral, physical or emotional – it's spiritual. In a new online survey by Beliefnet. 55% say sex is at least a part of their spiritual lives, with fully one third reporting: "my sexuality is an integral part of my spirituality"; 38% say they have prayed before or after sex, and 48% primarily define sex as a gift from God." … 51% of men say that sex is primarily "a gift from God…

Beliefnet.com, in Newsweek Oct 2 2006

We have all the theories, systems, manifestoes, programs, ideas, insights, visions and agendas that we need to create a new and better world, but we still keep getting things wrong. This is because most of the human beings who are trying to apply these theories, systems etc. have low to middling BLOBs. Capitalism, for example, could be a perfectly fair just system guaranteeing a decent education, opportunities and lifestyle for everyone, but when many successful capitalists are low BLOB people who have no wish to share what they have, no wish to help the poor or disadvantaged better themselves, then the version we see of capitalism is harsh and inhuman.

How do we make better people?

You know the answer. Go to it, my friends.

God be with you both.

CONCLUSIONS

"I love you Patricia." It's the first time he's said it. Such a beautiful spring day. They're walking hand-in-hand around Descanso Gardens in Pasadena. Massed beds of roses are gleaming in the sun. On the other side of the trees ducks are splashing and quacking.

"**I** love you!*" She's laughing at him a little.*
"*I mean it!*"
She turns to look at him. They stand close. She's gazing into his eyes.
"*You love me, huh?*"
"*Yeah.*"
She nods.
"*Okay. I believe you. *"
"*So… Patricia…. I mean…. come on….!*"
"*What?*"
"*Do you love me?*"
"*Oh. Right. Do I love you?*"
She smiles into his eyes, then looks away at the roses. Glossy white, rich deep red.
"*I just wanna let it grow Mick. In its…*"
"*Yeah but…*"

"I can't say yes, and I can't say no. Yet."

"So what can you say?"

"I can say… Let's go check out the lake!"

He takes his hand away and stands there on the path. She walks on a few steps then stops and looks back at him. He gazes away across the flower – beds. He's, what? He's annoyed, or sulky. Wants more than he's getting. Wants to know where he stands. Wants to feel that he's on top of what's going on. Wants her, Patricia.

He takes a deep breath, turns back and they look at one another. All the questions and the comments and the me me me voices fade away. It's all here, everything they want. He reaches out his hand to her. She walks back and takes it.

Most of us are getting married in our mid-twenties, so we have at least a decade to go before we are – from the traditional, religious viewpoint – "allowed" to go to bed with one another. Expecting young people to wait ten or more years and to be celibate all that time, is clearly unrealistic. "So what are we supposed to do?" asked a college student one day when we were talking about this. " I think you have to work things out for yourself," was my answer. She gave me that "Copout!" look, and I think she was right to. Now, if the question was asked, my short, straight-from-the-shoulder, take it or leave it answer would be:

"Don't sleep around. Don't do hook-ups. Don't have sex when you're drunk or stoned. Don't have sex just so that he or she will like you. Don't have sex just because everyone else is. Even if you really like the person, or love him or her, don't jump into bed straight away. Get to know one another. Enjoy one another's company for a while. Stay in touch with, and listen to, your deeper feelings, or your inner voice. If it really feels right for you to make love together, don't settle for a quickie in the back of the car or in the bathroom of someone's

house during a crazy party. Let everything be right. And, if you can, say a prayer inside you or together, for your lovemaking to be blessed with love and tenderness as well as passion."

This book is the long answer. The most satisfying – to me – comment about it came from a hairdresser named Gabrielle who read it and said, " *Yes, well, this is what nearly everyone thinks Emmanuel.* " I hope that "Loving" reminds you of truths you already know, and that you found yourself looking up from the page from time to time and nodding, recognizing an insight you've already had, a truth you've already sensed, even if you hadn't put it into words. I'd rather remind you of a truth you already know than tell you a truth you've never thought of before.

Whatever's true in "Loving" is discovered, not invented.

Neither I nor anyone else has the right to be your teacher. Your inner, or your spirit – which is there within you waiting for you to start looking for it, waiting to come to life – is your teacher. You were born with everything you need to live in this world, including the understanding of what's right for you and what's harmful, and the freedom to choose between the two.

May it be that, having read this book, you are able to make more conscious choices about your sex life.

I sincerely ask your forgiveness for anything I've said that hurt or offended you.

Appendix

This final section contains a couple of chapters that are more academic in content.

1. The Life Energies

The ability to see the Great Truth of the hierarchic structure of the world, which makes it possible to distinguish between higher and lower Levels of being, is one of the indispensable conditions of understanding. Without it, it is not possible to find out where everything has its proper and legitimate place.

— Fritz Schumacher

I've talked a lot about "higher" and "lower" energies in this book. This section, I hope, will throw some light on these terms. There's an old guessing game called: 'Animal, vegetable, mineral. ' Sometimes we play it on long car journeys. Add 'human' and we have four levels, or energies. These four energies were once called 'The Great Chain of Being', and they provided a framework, or paradigm that, for centuries, shaped our understanding of life. Some version of The Great Chain is found in many cultures.

Everything in the world is the expression of one of these four energies, and it's important to understand that they are not only *out there*, in the world, but *in here*, in our beings. In the complete Great Chain there are seven energies; the top three are 'perfect human', 'angelic', and 'prophetic'. It's the four lower ones we're looking at here. You can, with a little practice, use these energies as a way to clarify BLOB. *Each energy contains the energies beneath it, plus a radically different force, or energy. All these four energies are present in our beings.*

Animal, material, vegetal, human. If you think about these energies you may be able to sort them out into a kind of table, or hierarchy. (Hierarchy, according to my dictionary, means 'a system of persons or things arranged in a graded order'. In other words, a system of classification that goes from lower to higher). Which do you think is the lowest? Which one is next? And next? Which one is at the top? So… here's a brief introduction to the life energies, starting at the bottom.

1. Material energy

The lowest is the material energy – water, metal, stone, glass, plastic, concrete, weapons, money etc. It's matter. It's been described as the 'floor' for all the other energies. It's passive and inert. It may seem dead, or inanimate, but, as scientists have discovered, in its own way it's alive, full of vibrations, or energy. A rock is made of tingling particles of energy.

Any structure it possesses is created by an outside, higher energy. So a computer is a material object that has been assembled by a human being. A tree is a life process in which material forces – sunlight, water, nutrients – are transformed by the vegetable force into a living form that grows, blossoms, bears fruit (seeds) and dies.

Without the material energy we'd be invisible. It gives us our fluids, our bones, our physical mass. Without it we'd have no buildings, no cars, no electricity or gas, no jet planes or roads. We'd have no rivers, no mountains, no wind or clouds or deserts. So the material energy is a vital part of our lives.

However, the material energy can influence our thinking and feeling and actions so strongly that it can take us over. People who are obsessed with gaining more and more money or possessions without caring whom they hurt in the process are in the grip of the material energy.

The material energy is currently very strong in the world. However, it's not that it's *wrong*. As we've seen, we can't live without it. *The issue is our relationship with it.* Nuclear energy, for example, can be used to provide us with power that enhances our lives, or it can be used to destroy millions of people. Money in itself has no value. Like nuclear power, it's neutral. It can be used to build better schools and provide adequate health care for everyone and to develop sources of power that do not harm the planet (and therefore our lives) or it can be used to build more and more powerful weapons whose purpose is to threaten or destroy other human beings.

What does this have to do with sex? The material energy can 'hitch a ride', as it were, on our sexuality. Here are some examples:

*When a prostitute exchanges sex for money, she's using her body as a material object.

*When a young man is raped in prison, men are using him as an object.

*When a couple have sex in front of film cameras for money, they are using themselves and one another as objects. They are doing what they are doing for money, so this is the content of their actions.

*When you get someone so drunk or so stoned that they don't know what's going on, and then have sex with them, you're using them as an object.

I saw a staged monolog in L.A. years ago in which a woman told the story of how a van bumped into the back of her car in the street at night. She got out to check the damage, and two men jumped out of the van and forced her into the back seat of her car. One kept watch while the other pulled out a knife and held it to her throat, and then began tearing at her clothes.

She didn't fight back. She didn't scream. She started talking to the man. She told him her name; she told him about where she grew up, about her parents and her brothers and sisters. She told him what she did, and what she did, and what her home was like. He told her to shut up, but she kept telling him about her life and about herself. Finally the man climbed off her, looked at her for a moment, swore, then got out of the car. The two men got in their van and drove away. *The woman had refused to be treated as an object.*

'Object' is material. 'It' is the material level pronoun. I had a friend years ago who was a real womanizer. Describing his sex life he said, "*I've poked a few things since then.*" Using another person's body as an object – pornography and prostitution – is sexuality that is filled with the material force.

2. Vegetable energy

If the material force is existence, the vegetable force is life. Sustenance is taken from the material level and is given life and form. Plants react to their environment – to light, to temperature, to moisture – and they compete with one another.

Clearly there's a jump in the chain as we move from material to vegetable, one that's a matter of KIND rather than DEGREE. If we call the material force 'm', and plants are v, then we get m+v. (Remember that forces contain the forces beneath them).

Plants could be called natural egotists. They go for what they need with no awareness of other plants. They are nothing but 'self'.

If we did not have the vegetable force within us, we could not eat. We could not live. The vegetable force maintains all those physical processes that we call 'involuntary' – our circulatory system, our digestion, our breathing, and so on. People in comas are sometimes described as being in a 'vegetative' state

'Feelings' – the immediate, up-and-down, reactive feelings – are vegetable.

While we're talking about the veggie energies I want to say something about drugs and alcohol. Please stay with me.

The material energy is very strong in our lives. Most of us live and work in concrete and glass boxes, travel around in metal boxes, belong to a society dominated by market forces, go through an educational system that is increasingly governed by test scores, spend a lot more time in rooms with computers than in woods full of birdsong and deer-prints. So the vegetable kingdom that drugs lift us to may feel, by comparison, like bliss. (It depends on your BLOB of course. A person with a human level of being will probably enter a state of deep spiritual panic if they get stoned.) Alcohol, heroin, cocaine and marijuana, all powerful carriers of the vegetal energy, provide an escape from the pressure of the material force. However, absorbing these plant forces into our psyches is harmful to us. If we become addicted we lose touch with our animal natures, and with our humanity. We become entities who look like human beings but whose content is no different from that of plants.

When you're stoned you can FEEL, you can have SENSATIONS. That's what plants do, in their own limited way. But also, when you're stoned you find it harder to make decisions, to think clearly, to remember facts, to relate to people who aren't stoned, to discriminate, to empathize with other people, to follow through and finish a project. Your sex drive will diminish and you may become paranoid. A central message of this book is that we are responsible for how we feel, what we think and what we do. This is what being human means. We can fulfill this responsibility only if we are fully conscious of what's going on within us and around us.

The following anecdote, taken from an extraordinary book: "Smashed", is a very accurate depiction of the displaced, not-really-here state induced by heavy drinking. It's Hallowe'en; they've been drinking in a graveyard: *Mac is heavier than he looks. When he lowers his skinny skater frame on top of me I feel like I'm being buried alive. I think of Madeline in the "Fall of the House of Usher" which we just read in school, and wonder at what point she stopped scratching the lid of the coffin and just fell into death, the way I let Mac fall into me. He is holding my head with both hands, the way I might hold an open book. My hat slides off and falls at the foot of Barker's tombstone, where someone bereft would place a bouquet. ..... At this moment I am not one bit chicken. I like the anonymity, the fact that I don't know who I'm kissing beneath his skeleton suit. Mac isn't kissing me either. He's kissing my shit face, which makes me feel less vulnerable... Mac is pressed smack into me. He is closer than any boy has ever been before, but I feel like there is a protective layer between us, a type of atmospheric safe sex.*

His tongue parts my lips. His breath is potent, the way I imagine mine must be, and his cold wet lips remind me of a bowl of eyeballs (they were really skinned grapes) I stuck my hand into once when I was blindfolded at a Halloween party. I kiss him back because out of the corner of my eye I see that Billie is kissing Phil, and that seems as good a reason as any. Mac's hands are on me too, latching on to me in places I myself don't dare touch. One curled hand is wrapped around the bantam bulge of my bra, the other kneading my upper, upper thigh like he is trying to give me a charley horse. I see where he's touching me more than I can feel it. My synapses are bootless beneath layers of thermal underwear and the deadening effect of brandy. I could be thumbed and needled and barely feel a thing. I try to will myself to reciprocate, but I can't find my hands. Thanks to apple brandy I can only gauge my general position. I can see the outline of my body as though I am watching myself from far away, the way people who've come back from the brink of death claim they watched doctors resuscitate them from high above their own operating tables. My body is there in the dirt, tucking one Herculean hand under the back of his T-shirt (it must be cold because it makes him shiver) while my essence is someplace much higher, far above the cigarette butts and the stone rows and the longest-reaching flashlight beams.[1].

If my sexuality is expressing the vegetable energy then the pleasure I experience is personal, enclosed, private. It's masturbation, self-sex, me-sex. D.I.Y. sex. It's a closed lonely loop. Masturbation isolates us, draws us ever more deeply into head-sex fantasies, and siphons off energy that is potentially very high and creative.

3. Animal energy

The animal energy would be m+v+a . What's the 'a' factor? What can we characterize as animal? We could include 'consciousness'. However we define it, we can surely recognize a kind of consciousness in a monkey or a dog. Clearly there's more consciousness, more complexity and more freedom in the life of an eagle than there is in the life of a rhubarb plant. Besides consciousness, animal characteristics include sexuality, group life, and territoriality/aggression.

We human beings have the animal energies in us. So we fight, we mate, we protect our young, we belong to families, communities, tribes, nations...and we may reject or attack members of other tribes or nations. We have strong social and survival instincts. We have rules, customs, taboos, many of which are based on survival. We engage in numerous struggles for power and dominance, whether in the marriage, the street gang, the high school campus, the board room, the political system or the U.N.

Animals are biologically conditioned. They have little or no freedom to make choices. They are conscious, but they are not aware of *themselves*. When we identify with a group and unthinkingly assimilate the group's attitudes: "We're the best!" "The Palestinians are sand niggers!" "Tree-hugger!" then we are expressing the animal force; we identify with a *part* of humanity – *'our'* part. On the other hand, the human energy moves us to identify with humanity, with all humankind. "God bless America" widens into "God bless the world." As, I believe, it will one day. It had better. It's our only chance of survival.

If we didn't have the animal energy in us, we wouldn't even recognize the opposite sex, let alone feel passion or sexual arousal. We wouldn't have the urge to mate, and to raise our children, so humanity as a species would die out.

For most of us, most of the time, sex is an expression of the animal energy. This is natural and normal.

But…. is it human?

4. Human energy

Let's have a look at the human energy before we try to answer this question.

We contain, we depend upon, we express, the material, vegetable and animal energies: m+v+a+h.. Each of these energies, except the material, contains those below it, plus a new, or radically different force, or energy.

A feature of the hierarchy is that there's a continual movement, or process of change going on, either up or down. Think, for example, of a hamburger:

Moisture and nutrients in the soil (material energies) are drawn through roots to become grass (vegetable) which is eaten by a cow and turned into meat (animal) which is eaten by a human being.

What is there that we can define as human, and therefore different to the three other energies? In particular, what makes us different to the animals?

Animals, when they experience a sexual urge, have no choice in the matter. They go for it. They mate, or they court or fight so that they can mate. We human beings, on the other hand, *have the capacity to postpone the gratification of our sexual impulses.* We may not want to postpone anything. We may just want to go ahead and do it. But we don't have to. *We can choose.* We can decide whether or not to go ahead.

This is a major difference. This ability to stand back from our desires and choose is a significant element in our humanity. In a way, it's one of the things that makes being human so hard, and, at the same time, so fulfilling. We know, deep down, that we always have a choice in what we do, and that we are therefore responsible for everything that we do. We have the freedom to choose whether or not to have sex.

It is precisely this freedom to choose that this book has been focusing on.

Another big difference between ourselves and animals is that they have seasons for their mating. With them, intercourse is clearly very closely linked to reproduction. They have sex in the mating season so that they can have babies and ensure the survival of their species. We, on the other hand, are sexually available almost all the time.

So, unlike animals, we have the choice to follow or not to follow our sexual impulses, and from puberty onwards this choice confronts us throughout the year. If, like most animals, we were sexually active only in the spring, then our lives would be very different.

We have this capacity to choose because, unlike animals, we're able to stand back and be self-aware. Also, we have the capacity to make sacrifices for the sake of an ideal or for an aim that's higher than our needs and appetites.

If we want to be true human beings, our task is to get to know the forces that are alive inside us, and – with help from a higher power, or a power within ourselves that we seek, nurture and learn to trust– learn to control them. This takes time. It's hard, hard work. But the growing sense of lightness and inner freedom that we experience as we journey towards true humanity makes it all worthwhile.

(For more insights into this topic, see: "Being Human", by Solihin and Alicia Thom and Alexandra ter Horst, Pub. by Ad Humanitas Press 2004, "A Guide for the Perplexed" by Fritz Schumacher, pub. by Perennial Press 1978, and "The Pattern of the World" by Salamah Pope, Hilltop Press 2007)

2. MALE AND FEMALE

*A man may lust after **women**, but a woman lusts after
a man.*

— Lillian. B. Rubin

For years there's been an ongoing discussion about
the psychological differences between males and
females. Some claim that these differences are
caused by social conditioning (nurture), others that
they're the result of biological elements: the male and
females brains, hormones and bio-chemistry (nature).
I believe the "nature" people are right and that male/
female differences are primarily the result of how we're
"wired", not of how we're brought up, although it has
to be said that social conditioning plays a major role in
our sex lives.

Thanks to their wiring, men are better at advanced
math involving abstract concepts of space and
relationships. They're better at ball sports, map-reading
and chess. Women are better at learning foreign
languages, singing in tune, at expressing themselves
through language, at picking up social cues from tone

of voice or facial expressions, and, because of this ability, judging character.

The ways men and woman respond emotionally reflect differences in brain structure and organization. Men's emotions are stored over on the right side of the brain and their ability to express these emotions in speech over on the *other* side. Since these two halves don't share much connecting fiber, the information flow between them is limited, making it harder for a man to express his emotions.

Both sides of the female brain have emotional capacities, and the connections between them are much more numerous, so language and emotion are more integrated, making it easier for women to experience and talk about their feelings, and to create intricate, intimate relationships. Women tend to want long-term bonds, men short-term sexual activity.

Here's an analysis by Salamah of the male and (especially) the female experience of puberty: …. *a boy has ejaculations from puberty, whether or not he masturbates and whether or not he has sexual experience with a girl. So he is a consciously sexual creature from the moment of his first emission. Whereas all that the menarche (onset of a girl's menstrual periods) does is to make her feel somewhat handicapped/afflicted and even somewhat inferior. In other words, puberty in a girl induces no consciousness of sexuality. Unconsciously, yes, the hormones of her body begin to prepare her for long-term motherhood, but this is a very different thing from the boy's immediate understanding of himself as a woman-hunter.*

One result of this biological difference is that whereas a boy at puberty is a highly sexual creature, a virginal girl is not. Her sexuality takes some time to awaken; that is, to rise up from the unconscious to the conscious. (And, very often it takes an interest in one particular male to do this – as distinct from the boy's interest in practically all girls)

In the meantime, before she is awakened sexually, a girl may be aware only that the physical menarche causes changes to happen in her feelings; she will become far less sure of herself, unstable, moody and even highly emotional as the hormones play havoc with her still latent sexuality.

This has further consequences. Once a girl's sexuality has been aroused, directed usually towards one particular man or boy, her hormones will stop messing up her feelings generally, and focus on coming close to the young man she has romantic feelings for. As this escalates, her previously dormant sexuality becomes more and more conscious.

Once a girl is aware of her own sexuality, her body (or rather, her hormonal drive complex) takes over. She may think she is making responsible choices.... but the chances are her decisions are actually made on the still unconscious basis of her hormones. She may, in other words, be deceiving herself. Or rather, her emotions may be leading her to make choices her rational mind would not approve... And the war between her head and her heart has begun.

In any case, once a girl has entered into a fully sexual relationship, she is a very different person from her original, virginal self . First, her sexuality, now fully awakened, brings her happiness and, for a while, contentment. Also, as we've seen, she has literally taken another person on board.

However, when this relationship ends, as most do, she is no longer capable of making clear and rational decisions. Why not? Because her body, having become used to a satisfactory sex life, wants more – and, behind the scenes her now frustrated hormones hold her emotional and mental life in thrall.

Now, being a woman I don't know this from my own experience, but I suspect that boys have less trouble detaching themselves from their feelings.

Let's list more of these gender differences:

Men are less in touch with their feelings because of the way their brains are wired. The male hormone, testosterone tends to direct males towards independence and aggression.

The female hormones – estrogen, progesterone and prolactin – influence women towards empathy and cooperation. Away from independence and towards intimacy.

How do these differences pan out in real life? One international survey found that men admire such qualities as shrewdness, competitiveness, domination, assertiveness, and self-control, while women admire affection, cooperation, spontaneity, sympathy and generosity. In another, men prioritized power, freedom, political and economic values, while women gave priority to personal relationships and security, and aesthetic and religious values. [1]

Because of their biological makeup, men have a natural desire for sexual novelty. This has been called 'The Coolidge Effect'.

President Coolidge and his wife were visiting a government farm. Passing the chicken coop, Mrs. Coolidge inquired how often the rooster copulated each day.

'Dozens of times,' was the reply. 'Please tell that to the President,' Mrs. Coolidge requested.

When the President passed the pens and was told about the rooster, he asked, 'Same hen every time?' 'Oh no Mr. President, a different one each time.' The President nodded slowly, then said, 'Tell that to Mrs. Coolidge.'

In addition to these biological/hormonal factors there's our human history. Before our shift to agriculture 10,000 years ago, we were, for millions of years, hunters and gatherers. Women birthed and cared for babies, looked after the "home" and participated in the local community, and gathered food, firewood etc, from nearby. Men sired offspring, formed and were part of larger alliances, and hunted.

To do their work, women needed to hear, touch, taste and smell and be aware of small physical details, (a child's whimper, an unseen edible root) and they needed to scan and respond to the emotive data from family or immediate community. They needed to be able to multi-task. Men needed an acute sense of dimensionality, depth perception and judgment of distance. To kill animals, fight other tribes and protect their community men needed strength, physical skill and aggression rather than empathy and communication skills. These different brains are with us still.

Life was harsh back then; the survival of the tribe required that men, like cockerels, impregnate as many females as they could.

Men find satisfaction in the sexual act itself, in the build-up to, and the experience of, orgasm. Women find satisfaction when sex is the expression of intimacy and tenderness. So while the man, assuming that the woman is a mirror image of himself, may be intent on *performance* – and that she therefore wants a man who can go at it like a supercharged bull – the woman wants to be gently stroked and intimately loved, not possessed as an object of skin and flesh. This need for sexuality as the expression of a secure and committed relationship may explain why women are 17 times more likely to experience orgasm in marriage than out of marriage.

One study quoted in 'Brain Sex' reports that college students were asked to evaluate their degree of sexual satisfaction on a 1–5 scale with a range of partners – casual acquaintances, friends, and lovers. Men scored sex with acquaintances at 4.2, with friends at 4.4, and with lovers at 4.9. Women rated sex with friends and with lovers as more or less the same as men. But they rated sex with acquaintances at only 1.0.

In view of these natural differences, why are thousands of young women choosing to act like men, and have casual sex? I came across a quote that touched me with its bleakness: *"Sometimes it's easier to have sex with a guy than talk to him."* Perhaps one of the less positive messages of feminism is that young women are free to – even expected to – behave like young men in the sexual arena. They are free to have casual sex. *"It's 1997, and chicks like unencumbered sex as much as men do."* (GQ Magazine)

It's as though we've been trying to pretend that there aren't really any basic differences between the sexes; it's all a matter of conditioning, of upbringing, of social pressures. We've been so caught up with political and social equality we've forgotten, or denied, biological and psychological diversity. But girls and young women – I believe – do violence to their femininity when they sleep with men they have no relationship with, men they may not even talk to, men they may not even *like*. They are suppressing the 'intimacy imperative', their innate need for love, affection, tenderness, intimacy, empathy, and friendship.

What about men? Is it okay for young men to go out and score as often as they can? To 'sow their wild oats', as the old phrase says. Let's consider this question carefully.

Remember the rooster who copulated several times a day, with different chickens? This is what cockerels do. The fact is, though, *men are not cockerels*. Men aren't animals. Yes, we have animal force in us. But our destiny is to be (or to become) *humans*, not animals.

It may be true that men's brains are structured so that they separate sex from emotions and are therefore able, like the cockerel, to enjoy sex with multiple partners. However, there's a flaw in this scenario. Obviously, it's not possible for men to do this unless there are available women. But we've seen that women aren't made that way.

Back when we were hunters and gatherers, for the sake of the survival of the species, men had to go around copulating with women. They had little or no choice in the matter. We might say, then, that they were living on the animal level.

As we evolved from our nomadic phase to our more settled, agriculturalist phase life became less dangerous. Infant mortality dropped, life expectancy increased. However, right up to the nineteenth century, most of us married for economic rather than personal, or romantic reasons. Big families meant more hands available to work the land. Because of the still relatively high rates of death in childbirth and of infant mortality, sex for most women was strongly linked to death. In 17th century Europe and America almost 25% of infants died in their first year. [2]

Put these factors together and it's reasonable to assume that intercourse for many was a somewhat brief and joyless affair, especially for women. Not much time for, or interest in, kissing, cuddling, whispering sweet nothings etc. In the nineteenth century, as the need for big families became less urgent, the economic basis for marriage gave way to that of romantic love.

So the biological imperative has become less urgent, although it was, up until quite recently, still paramount. We might say that sex has changed from being a brief functional rutting to be an experience that could be enjoyed for itself, a change given further momentum by the condom and the pill. We might say that sex has been *feminized*. We might say that, *potentially*, our behavior has moved from the animal survival level to the human level.

History has given us choice, one of its greatest and most challenging gifts.

Let's go back to rampant male lust. Can it be checked? Can a man learn to control it? The answer, obviously, is Yes. Men are controlling their sexual urges all the time. If men followed every sexual impulse they experience, society as we know it would disintegrate.

Take a moment to visualize....

.... a shopping mall on a busy Saturday. Steve and his mates Finn and Jose walk in through the entrance. There's a beautiful young woman standing outside Victoria's Secret, talking on her cell phone. Long dark hair, sleek black skirt, white blouse.

Steve pauses briefly, checks around for her mate, sees none, advances on her, growling deeply. Meanwhile Finn has been checking her out. Jose's off after another female he saw going into the Body Shop. Steve sniffs the air, smells Finn's pheromones, snarls at him. Finn bares his teeth and snarls back. Steve grabs a handful of Finn's hair. They're snarling and smashing at one another. The girl whimpers, slinks back into the boutique and hides behind a display of black negligees.....

Unlike animals – and our distant ancestors – we can and do delay the gratification of our desires, a capacity that defines us as *human.*

What does it mean to be a man? I don't believe it means scoring as many girls as we can. We may fantasize about having her and also having her, having the cheerleader with creamy thighs, the girl with big boobs behind the coffee-bar counter, the blonde in the black bikini sunbathing on the beach a few yards away ... but serial sexuality, while in line with our primitive script, gratifying to the ego and pleasurable, is an abuse of our beings.

Here's what I believe. DON'T REACT PLEASE … Read, feel, ponder…

The man is the channel through which a new life comes into the world. He is the source of the human seed, of the children who will follow him and take the future into their hands after he is gone. If he has sex with multiple partners, especially with women who have been promiscuous, then he will bring the destructive effects of this behavior into the union between himself and his wife, and she will suffer spiritually as a result.

And what of the child they may one day conceive? If a man sleeps around a lot then gets married and becomes a father, how will his experiences affect the child's inner? Here's an insight from the Javanese sage, Pak Subuh:

"So, later on, when he begets a child, his child will also be swayed by those lower forces… Because of this, the child will eventually have to suffer a great deal in his life, especially in becoming aware of his human identity. The reason is that almost the whole content of the child's inner feeling has been affected by the lower forces, thus causing his thoughts always to be directed to the interests of those forces." [3]

So the man has some significant choices to make. Potentially, he is the bringer of order, the source of reason and rightness, the one who discriminates between lust and love, this impulse and that impulse. The sword of the noble knight symbolizes this capacity to discriminate. Ideally, when the man feels sexual desire he will know its source and its quality. He'll be able to choose whether to act on it or not. A man who is in control of his sexuality will be very attractive to his partner. She will feel and respond to his inner strength. There's a deep contest going on between the sexes. If he can't keep his hands off her he's lost.

David, an English friend, once asked me: "*Can you watch a sexy scene in a movie without being aroused?*"

I thought about it. "*No, I don't think I can.*"

He nodded. "*Huh.*"

"*What do you mean... Huh?*"

"*Nothing.*"

I was getting annoyed.

"*Come on...*"

He wouldn't say any more. That was his style. Enigmatic. But for some reason I kept thinking about his question, and his "Huh". And then, it must have been at least two years later, I was watching a movie; a fairly steamy scene was playing... and I consciously withdrew from my involvement. I observed, but held myself separate. "*I'm not going to let this turn me on.*" And I wasn't aroused. Sat there in the flickering gloom thinking Wow.

What was the point? Simply this: I wanted to be able to exercise some control over my responses. *No, I don't want that feeling in me.* I was learning to discriminate. The ruler is back where he belongs and the servants are in their places.

An important part of the journey that a relationship takes us on is, for the man, the recognition and acceptance of the female element in his nature, (the 'anima', as Jung calls it) and, for a woman, a corresponding recognition of her male element (the animus). If the man has learnt to live comfortably with the feminine part of himself, then he can live comfortably and in peace with a woman, and vice versa. Recently I was looking at a painting of a weird squadron of murderous-looking politicians streaking through the sky. Below them bombs were bursting among crowds of panic-stricken people. It was a powerful image, one that still haunts me. The painter, Leonard Lasalle, told me: "*This is a painting of men who have lost touch with their feminine aspects. If we want a peaceful world, men have to find the woman in themselves. It may be easier to do this than to find God.*"

Here's a list of masculine and feminine qualities:

Masculine
Penetration
Discrimination
Adventurousness
Discipline
Competitiveness

Feminine
Receptiveness
Protectiveness
Nurturing
Endurance
Pragmatism
Co-operation

Jungian writer Robert Johnson says that if we men are going to "be all that we can be" we must go through two stages in our relationship with our anima, or internal female nature:

1 Learn to control her, so that we are no longer swayed by her moods – sulks, irrational outbursts, etc.
2 Once this is done, learn to relate to her as an inner friend who brings warmth, tenderness and empathy to our lives. She can love us, if we let her. [4]

REFERENCES

How having sex affects us.
(1) Soul of Sex
By Thomas Moore
Pub. by Harper Collins 1998
Pp. 13 and 147

Fields
(1) Natural Grace,
by Rupert Sheldrake,
Pub. Doubleday 1996
p. 101

Basic Levels of Being
(1) Susila Budhi Dharma
By Muhammad-Subuh Sumohadiwidjojo
Pub. by Subud Publications International 1975
p. 305

Sex in the Head
(1) The Beauty Myth
By Naomi Wolf
Pub. by William Morrow and Co. NY 1991
p. 79

(2) The Way We Never Were
By Stephanie Coontz
Pub. by Basic Books
A division of Harper Collins Publishers 1992
p. 199
(3) Pornotopia
by Rick Poynor
Pub. by Princeton Architectural Press
N.Y. 2006
p. 136
(4) Sex Violence and Pornography
By Susan G. Cole
Pub by Second Story Press
1995
pp. 75, 76
(5) Ways of Seeing
By John Berger
Pub. by Penguin Books USA 1977
p. 47

Being the Boss
(1) Emotional Intelligence
by Daniel Goleman
Pub. by Bloomsbury Publishing 1996
p. 80
(2) Social Intelligence
by Daniel Goleman
Pub. by Bantam Books 2006
Pp 63- 82

The Choice
(1) Why can't we be good?
by Jacob Needleman

Pub. by Jeremy P. Tarcher/Penguin
2007
p. 13

Who am I?
(1) Why can't we be good?
by Jacob Needleman

Pub. by Jeremy P. Tarcher/Penguin
2007
p. 9

The Vacuum
(1) Make Peace with Anyone
by David J. Lieberman
pub. St Martins Press 2002
p. 6

The Law of Cosmic Balance
(1) Helen Merrell Lynd
On Shame and the Search for Identity
Quoted in: Teens Under the Influence
By Katherine Ketcham and Nicholas A. Pace MD
Ballantine Book pub. By Random House Publishing
Group
2003
p. 233

Abortion
(1) Aborted Women
by David Readon
pub. by University of Loyola Press 1987
p. 130
(2)Embraced by the Light
By Betty J. Eadie
Pub. Gold Leaf Press 1992
P. 95 p. 97

The Life Forces
(1) Smashed
by Koren Zailckas
Pub by Penguin Books
2005
Pp 47, 48

Male and Female
(1) Brain Sex
By Anne Moir and David Jessel
Pub. Dell Publishing
Bantam Doubleday Dell Publishing Group Inc.
N.Y 1991
P. 130
(2) The Transformation of Intimacy
by Anthony Glidden
Pub. by Stanford University Press 1992
pp. 27, 38, 39.
(3) Susila Budhi Dharma
By Muhammad-Subuh Sumohadiwidjojo
Pub. By Subud Publications International 1975
p. 315
(4) "He" by Robert A. Johnson
Published by Perennial Library
Harper and Row 1974
p. 33

BIBLIOGRAPHY

(An asterisk * indicates recommended)
Abbott, Elizabeth. A History of Celibacy. Scribner, 2000.
Arredia, Joni. Sex, Boys and You. Perc Publishing, 1999.
*Barber, Benjamin R. Consumed. W.W.Norton 2007
Barash, David P. and Nanelle R. Madame Bovary's Ovaries. Bantam Dell, 2005
Bennett, J.G. Sex. Samuel Weiser Inc., 1981.
Berger, John. Ways of Seeing Penguin Books USA 1977
*Biddulp, Steve. Manhood. Finch Publishing, 1994.
Blake, Jeanne. Risky Times – A Guide for Teenagers. Workman Publishing Company, 1990.
Bly, Robert. Iron John. Addison-Wesley, 1990.
Bly, Robert, Hillman, James and Meade, Michael. The Rag and Bone Shop of the Heart. Harper Collins, 1992.
*Bonheim, Jalaja. Aphrodite's Daughters. Fireside Book, Simon and Schuster, 1997.
Bourgeault, Cynthia. Love is Stronger Than Death. Lindisfarne Books, 2001.

Bouris, Karen. The First Time. Conari Press Books, 1990.

*Bradley, Michael Bradley and O'Connor, Carroll. Yes Your Teen is Crazy. Harbor Press, 2001.

Branden, Nathaniel. The Psychology of Romantic Love. Bantam Books, 1983.

*Brown, Gabrielle. The New Celibacy. McGraw-Hill, 1980.

Bull, David. Cool and Celibate? Element Children's Books, 1998.

Campbell, Joseph. Creative Mythology. Viking Press, 1968.

Chandler, Sarah. Ophelia Speaks. Harper Collins Publishers Inc., 1999.

*Cole, Susan G. Sex, Violence and Pornography. Second Story Press, 1995.

*Coontz, Stephanie. American Families and the Nostalgia Trap. Basic Books, 1993.

Covey, Sean. The 7 Habits of Highly Effective Teens. Fireside, 1998.

*Crompton,Vicki and Zelda Kessner, Ellen. Saving Beauty from the Beast. Little Brown and Company, 2003.

*Davis Kasl, Charlotte. Women, Sex and Addiction. Harper and Row, 1989.

de Angelis, Barbara. What Women Want Men to Know. Hyperion, 2001.

de Angelis, Barbara. What Women Want You to Know. Hyperion, 2001.

de Rougemont, Denis. Passion and Society. Translated by M. Belgion. Faber and Faber Ltd., 1956.

Di Prisco, Joseph and Riera, Michael. Field Guide to the American Teenager. Perseus Publishing, 2002.

*Dines, Gail, Jensen, Robert and Ann Russo. Pornography – The Production and Consumption of Inequality. Routledge, 1998.

Eadie, Betty. Embraced by the Light. Gold Leaf Press, 1992.

*Ehrenreich, Barbara. Dancing in the Streets, Metropolitan Books, 2006.

Fein, Ellen and Schneider, Sherrie. The Rules. Warner Books, 1995.

Fischer, Norman. Taking Our Places. Harper San Francisco, 2003.

Fox, Matthew. One River, Many Wells. Penguin/Putman, 2000.

*Fromm, Erich. The Art of Loving. Harper and Row, 1956

Gilligan, Carol. The Birth of Pleasure. Alfred A. Knopf, 2002.

Gilmore, David, Mack, Dana and Nock, Steven. Marriage in the Making? – Report on the Courtship Customs of Young Americans. Institute for American Values, (undated).

*Glenn, Norval and Marquardt, Elizabeth – Principal Investigators. Hooking Up, Hanging Out, and Hoping for Mr. Right – College Woman on Dating and Mating Today. Institute for American Values, 2001.

*Glidden, Anthony. The Transformation of Intimacy. Stanford University Press, 1992

*Goleman, Daniel. Emotional Intelligence. Bloomsbury Publishing, 1996.

*Guerain, Michael. The Wonder of Boys. Jeremy P. Tarcher / Putnam, 1997.

*Guerian, Michael. The Wonder of Girls. Atria Books, 2002.

Hawken, Paul. The Ecology of Commerce. Harper Collins, 1993.

*Hendrix, Harville. Keeping the Love You Find: A guide for singles. Pocket Books, 1992.

*Hendrix, Harville. Getting the Love You Want. Simon and Schuster, 1993.

Irvine, Janice M. Talk About Sex. University of Califonia Press, 2002.

*Johnson, Robert. He. Perennial Press – Harper and Row, 1974.

*Johnson, Robert. We. Harper Collins, 1983.

*Johnson, Robert. She. Harper Perennial, 1989.

*Kantor, David. My Lover, Myself: Self-Discovery Through Relationship. Riverhead Books, 1999.

*Kas, Charloot Davis. Women, Sex and Addiction. Harper Row, 1989.

Kass, Amy A and Leon R. Eds: Wing to Wing Oar to Oar. Pub. by University of Notre Dame 2000

Kelly, Joe. Dads and Daughters. Broadway Books, 2002.

Ketcham, Katherine and Pace, Nicholas A. Teens Under the Influence. Ballantine Books. 2003.

Lattin, Don. Following our Bliss. Harper Collins Publishers Inc., 2003.

*Lengel, Beverly. The Right to Innocence. Ballantine Books, 1989.

Lerman, Evelyn. Safer Sex – The New Morality. Morning Glory Press, 2000.

Levy, Ariel. Female Chauvinist Pigs. Free Press 2006

Lewis, C.S. The Four Loves. Harcourt Brace and World Inc, 1960.

Liberman, David J. Make Peace with Anyone. St. Martins Press, 2002.

Mander, Jerry. In the Absence of the Sacred. Sierra Books, 1991.

Michael, Robert T., Gagnon, John H., Laumann, Edward O., and Kolata, Gina. Sex in America. Little Brown and Co., 1994.

Miller, Alice. For Your Own Good. H. and H. Hannum. Farrar Straus Giroux, 1983.

*Moir, Anne and Jessel, David. Brain Sex. Dell Publishing, 1991.

*Moore, Thomas. Soul of Sex. Harper Collins, 1998.

Needleman, Jacob Why can't we be good? Jeremy P. Tarcher/Penguin 2007

Orenstein, Peggy. Schoolgirls. Doubleday, 1994.

*Paul, Pamela, Pornified. Owl Books. 2006

Peck, Scott. The Road Less Traveled. Simon and Schuster Inc., 1978.

*Pipher, Mary. Reviving Ophelia. Grosset/Putnam, 1994.

*Pollack, William. Real Boys. Random House Inc., 1998.

*Pollak, William S. with Shuster, Todd. Real Boys' Voices. Penguin Books, 2000.

Pomeroy, Wardell B. and Haeberle, Erwin J. The Complete Guide to Safer Sex. The Institute for Advanced Study of Human Sexuality, (undated).

Ponton, Lynn. The Sex Lives of Teenagers. Penguin Putnam Inc., 2000.

Pope, Arthur Abdullah. Reminiscences of Bapak. Pub. Hilltop Farm Press, Perth Australia. 2005

Pope, Salamah. Sex and Sadness. Unpublished monograph, 2000.

*Pope, Salamah The Pattern of the World Pub. Hilltop Press 2007

Postman, Neil. Disappearance of Childhood. Delacorte Press, 1982.

Potts, Malcolm and Short, Roger. Ever Since Adam and Eve. Cambridge University Press, 1999.

Quart, Alissa. Branded. Perseus Press, 2003.

Ray, Paul H. Ray and Anderson, Sherry Ruth. Cultural Creatives. Harmony Books, 2000.

*Readon, David. Aborted Women. University of Loyola Press, 1987.

Rifkin, Jeremy, The European Dream. Jeremy P. Tarcher/Penguin. 2004

*Rilke, Rainer Maria. On Love and Other Difficulties. Translated by J.L. Mood. W.W.Norton and Co., 1975.

*Roffman, Deborah. Sex and Sensibility. Perseus Publishing, 2001.

Roiphe, Katie, The Morning After. Pub. by Little, Brown and Co. 1994

*Roiphe, Katie. Last Night in Paradise. Vintage Books, Division of Random House Inc., 1997.

*Rubin, Lillian B. Intimate Strangers. Harper and Row, 1983.

*Rubin, Lilian B. Erotic Wars. Farra Strauss and Giroux, 1990.

Rue, Nancy. Coping With Dating Violence. Rosen Publishing Co., 1989.

Ruiz, Don Miguel. The Four Agreements. Amber-Allen Publishing, 1997.

Schlosberg, Suzanne, The Curse of the Singles Table, Pub. by Warner Books 2004

*Schumacher, Franz. A Guide for the Perplexed. Perennial Press, 1978.

*Shalit, Wendy. A Return to Modesty. The Free Press, Division of Simon and Schuster, 1999.

*Shalit, Wendy, Girls gone mild, Random House, 2007

Shary, Timothy. Generation Multiplex. University of Texas Press, 2002.

Sheldrake, Rupert. Natural Grace. Doubleday, 1996.

Steyer, James P. The Other Parent. Atria Books, 2002.

Stoltenberg, John. The End of Manhood. Plume (an imprint of Dutton Signet), 1994.

Stoltenberg, John. Refusing to be a Man. Penguin Books, 1990.

Sumohadiwidjojo, Muhammed Subuh. Susila Budhi Dharma. Translated by Sharif Horthy. Subud Publications International, 1999.

Sunstein, Cass. Why Societies Need Dissent. Harvard University Press, 2003.

Tacey, David. The Spirituality Revolution. Harper Collins (Australia), 2003.

Thom, Solihin and Alicia, and der Horst, Alexander. Being Human. Ad Humanitas Press, 2004.

*Tolman, Deborah L. Dilemmas of Desire. Harvard University Press, 2002.

*Trachtenberg, Peter. Casanova Complex. Pocket Books – Simon and Schuster Inc., 1998.

*Turnbull, Colin M. The Human Cycle. Simon and Schuster, 1983.

Watson, Curtis Brown. Shakespeare and the Renaissance Concept of Honor. Princeton University Press, 1960.

Western, Carol. Girltalk about Guys. Perennial Library, 1988.

White, Emily. Fast Girls. Scribner, 2002.

Whitehead, Barbara Dafoe and Poppenoe, David. Should We Live Together? National Marriage Project, 2001.

*Whitehead, Barbara Dafoe and Poppenoe, David. The State of our Unions. National Marriage Project, 2002.

Wickes, Frances G. The Inner World of Childhood. Prentice Hall, 1965.

Williamson, Marianne. Illuminata: A Return to Prayer. Random House, 1994.

*Wolf, Naomi. The Beauty Myth. William Morrow and Co.,1991.

Youngs, Betty B. Helping Your Teenager Deal With Stress. Jeremy P. Archer Inc., 1986

.— Male and Female Rights and Responsisbilities in a Dating Relationship. New Jersey Dept. of Community Affairs – Division on Women, the Office on the Prevention of Violence against Women. (date?)

.— Reaching and Teaching Teens to Stop Violence. Nebraska Domestic Violence Assault Coalition, (date?)

.— Teenage Sexuality: Opposing Viewpoints. Edited by T.L.Roleff. Greenhaven Press, Inc., 2001

.— The Sexual Revolution. Edited by M. E. Williams. Greenhaven Press, 2002.

.— Transforming a Rape Culture. Edited by E. Buchwald, P. Fletcher, and M. Roth. Milkweed Editions, 1993.

You can find out about Subud by
Googling the name.
I recommend the website whatissubud.net